"When illness knocks on our door it can either destroy us and take us deeper into a vortex of negative emotions or as it is in Susan's case, it can become the greatest gift and the teacher that opens our wings required for us to rise from the ashes and fly like phoenix into new healthy horizons. In each chapter you will find nuggets of wisdom that truly help you embrace your strengths, innate abilities, and the healing power that gratitude, speaking your truth, and unconditional love can bring into your life. This book is a must read for those seeking the clarity required to take back the rains of their life and learn to make the choices required to help them on their journey to attain the balance required to achieving perfect health."

TONY J. SELIMI INTERNATIONAL BEST-SELLING AUTHOR, SPEAKER AND HUMAN BEHAVIOURAL EXPERT KNOWN AS THE SEE-THROUGH COACH

"A book written from the heart – Sue is open about her journey and allows us to experience the difficulties that both her and fellow dyslexics deal with on a daily basis. Having known Sue since she was about 12 years old I realise how well she hid the problems she faced and did her upmost to enjoy life and achieve what many people only dream about. Her tenacity and honesty is unmeasured and I thank her for her love and friendship."

SARAH ARMSTRONG - CRANIAL PRACTITIONER

CW00829749

"What a wonderful, wonderful book - I loved it! You won't believe I've just demolished it, cover to cover, there was no putting it down. I cried & laughed & loved the wisdom in it. The style was magic - so beautifully natural, refreshing, honest. Full of love."

KATE PETERS

This is a wonderful, authentic book which everyone can take something from. Sue has an amazing life force which she has used to turn life's potential disasters in to triumphs. She shares her inspiring story in a fun and accessible way. There are so many tips for making life better - make sure you read this book!

SARAH SPELLER A DEAR FRIEND

No SUGAR

My journey my choice

Sue Bannister

My route to

SELF RECOVERY – SELF IMPROVEMENT

Coincides with the news of having secondary cancer

Ian
Dear friend
thank you for always
being there, and
your calmers &
fun you bring
to my life
x M Bannister
Sue 24/10/2016

First Edition published 2016 by
(Your Publishing details, website or email address)

Copyright © Sue Bannister 2016
The right of Sue Bannister to be identified as the
author of this work has been asserted by her in
accordance with the Copyright, Designs and Patents
Act 1988

A CIP catalogue record for this book is available
from the British Library
ISBN 978-0-9955426-0-0

Dear Peter

I dedicate the book to you my husband
and soul mate.

with unconditional love
your dearest wife

Time line

1960   - April 12 born

1964   - First summer at Hayling Island Sailing Club

1965   - Nightmare started first school

1971/2   - Nuns singled me out and bullied me

1973/5   - February headmaster drunk
- Travel to Scotland every weekend to be a ski Instructor
- Handed in first homework B+

1976   - Left school for better opportunities
- Sponsored to ski with local Italian ski club

1979   - First introduced to Chamonix

1980/1   - Survived the era of extreme skiing in Chamonix
- Completed in the Ski Derby on Grant Montet first overseas team
- Choose a different path to Ronald's proposal

1982   - Private ferry to Cowes

1991/92 - Winter in Maribel skiing

1993/93 - Mature student Business and French Studies

1998   - Bought Hayling House

1999   - Set up own events business
- Married love of my life Peter

2000   - Madrid an event with challenges

2001   - Farewell to Daddy and whittling

2005   - Worked for Lord's during the Ashes
        - Peter's 50th Garden party
        - Family world tour

2009   - 600 mile cycle from Innverness to Petersfield

2011   - President of the British Isles Flying
          Fifteen Association
        - KPI 30 week accelerator programme

2012   - Managed the Austrian Olympic and
          Paralympics National House
        - Late September diagnosed with Breast cancer
        - Late September started chemotherapy
          8 cycles

2013   - February Operation to have local excision of
          right breast and auxilary node clearance
        - April commenced radiotherapy
        - Following by 12 months course of the
          Herceptin drug
        - September holiday to La Manga with friends

2014   - January family ski trip to Courchevel
        - July a week in Port Grimaud with Diana
        - Autumn made a promise to look after
          myself to my best ability
        - October diagnosed with second cancer right
          breast, white dot in left lung
        - Christmas in Wengan
        - December PDG PET/CT scan to the left lung
        - Farewell to Mummy, the best cake maker

2015   - January operation bronchoscopy & left
            VATS single port apical lower segmentectory
            of left lung, remove cancer from the left
            lower lung
           - March commenced 4 cycles of chemotherapy
           - April first session with Tony J. Selimi
           - June holiday to La Manga with friends
           - June surgery DIEP flap conjunction with
            mastectomy
           - August trip to Brittney coast
           - September trip to Sete south of France

2015   - November long weekend trip to Edinburgh

2016   - 22nd January Oncologist said I was clear of
            cancer yippee
           - January weeks skiing in Chatel with friends

About the Author Sue Bannister

I was born in the era of flower power and free milk at school; hardship was ending and entering into prosperity. My parents' passion for sailing engulfed the likes of myself and my two sisters. I spent most of my time around boats or bobbing around on the Solent with the family. Forging lifetime friendships at the age of 5, jumping in a cadet as a crew at Hayling Island Sailing Club, I was petrified and excited at the same time.

1965 My summers were magical and I loathed the start of September. Being dyslexic school wasn't my favourite pastime. However I found happiness with friends in the playground or joining in sports such as netball and hockey which I captained. It was great being a part of a team. At Portchester Secondary School, having introduced the school to skiing I went on the ski trip which I thoroughly enjoyed. I still tell the tale of how I got the head master drunk, just so we could all stay up late one night. During this time I was bullied, categorised and singled out as different to others. I left school unable to read and write properly with the same qualifications as Rodney Trotter, 'Only Fools and Horse's', GCSE in metal work, art and geography. Happy to put that behind me, I headed to the mountains with my love of skiing.

I believed at an early age 'the purpose of life' was to grow up, be an adult and get a job. But I remember my nephew once saying when we were buying some tickets for the local swimming baths at Guildford "no she is not an adult yet, she's not married". I was 25 at the time. I loved the way he judged I was still a child. Well strangely I had to agree with him, it took me until my late 30's to settle. After many winters' skiing in the Alps, travelling was very much in my veins. Possibly I never settled because I was still in search of my purpose. Sailing, skiing, cycling were my three loves until Peter came into my life. He brought new meaning to passion for me.

My years of work at various companies had a common thread, looking after individuals or groups in one form or other. I was soon recognised for understanding and managing processes and brought in as a troubleshooter for some large organisations to deliver their events. But I never seemed to get the right break in my mind's eye in those early years at work.

With that in mind in my mid 30's I embarked on an access for business and finance course with the intention to do a degree in hotel management. Fortunately I was advised this wasn't the right path for me, and enrolled on a vocational course instead. I qualified with a merit in HNC business with French studies, yes French. This was a great turning point in my life; I was more measured and balanced. Over the next couple of years I moved into management with a small agency and worked at Marylebone Cricket Club. However I didn't seem settled working at them. I felt they were missing the mark, so my own events management company took shape, which allowed me to employ 5 team members, buying a share of boat the a flying fifteen and an office in Petersfield.

Just before turning 40 my two lifelong dreams came true. I bought a house and married the man I love, Peter. The past 17 years have been so amazing, he's not only been my partner, helm and soul mate, I am surprised how each year we have grown closer together. He has this incredible gift of pulling special moments out of a hat. I have been so spoilt I hear other partners commenting how lucky I am, "it is OK, I know I am." I am looking forward to many more lovely surprises in the next 40 plus years.

I have done some crazy things, sailing, skiing and cycling those adventures will have to wait for my next book or books. Do ask me if you want to hear more. Surviving the extreme era skiing in Chamonix, cycling from Inverness to Petersfield in the depths of winter and then more recently taking the role of the President of the British Isles International Flying Fifteen Association gave me little time for quietness.

Looking for clear direction and new goals to achieve and still looking for my purpose in my early 50's I found myself enrolled on a business accelerator programme. It was challenging, rewarding, hard and scary. I remember how awful I was at pitching on pitch fest day. What a great wake-up call to understand and to recognise the need for a perfect pitch, thank you. It was fantastic; I still keep in touch with some people from the course. I was amazed how it opened my eyes to new ideas and taught me to pitch and present, the tools I still use today.

I have had some great projects. Possibly my highlight to date was in 2012 being assigned to support The Corporation of Trinity House by managing the Austrian Olympic and Paralympics National House in London. Everyone involved truly embraced their role; it was a great example of partnerships working at their best from internal teams to border control. It was an amazing opportunity, a privilege and such fun to be involved.

The friends in the sailing world and Hayling Island have played a very big part in my life and I feel blessed to have such a bond with friends. The great things are the little things of knowing my neighbours for over 50 years or planning and organising the club quiz with Sue Moss for the past 12 years which has been a total hoot. My role is MC and I am responsible for the quiz rules, format and challenges! As the night unfolds the competitors have to create one of my wacky challenges, over the years they have made Wallace and Gromit, build a Thunderbird 2, create the magic roundabout and this year dressed up as Bernie the racing ostrich; God knows what they are going to make next year. It is hilariously funny and for a great cause, last year we designated it to memory of Bev Moss, Sue's beloved husband, raising over £1200 for cancer research.

In the autumn of 2012 aged 52 my journey took an uncertain turn. Suffering from tenderness in my right breast, inverted nipple, and stiffening under my right armpit, the latter restricting the movement of that arm, my doctor was quick to refer me to The Royal Marsden Rapid Diagnostic and Assessment Centre. I was first diagnosed with grade "3 DCIS 56 mm of the right breast triple negative and lymph node positive on right arm pit." I immediately started a course of neo-adjuvant EC-taxol after being diagnosed, the chemotherapy was brutal, my immune system went dangerously low causing me to be hospitalised on 3 occasions during the 7 cycles of treatment.

When I became unwell from the brutal treatment, I scaled down my work only taking on assignments that fitted around my treatment. I have been so fortunate to work on the Harrison's Fund charity Sky High Ball which has opened my eyes to Duchenne, a charity that deserves support and investment equal to that which breast cancer charities receive.

In February 2013 the team at the Royal Marsden Sutton operated, carrying out a local excision and auxiliary node clearance. They went on to give me a course of adjuvant radiotherapy with concomitant boost and right supraclavicular fossa which was under the guidance of the IMPORT High study, followed by eighteen cycles of adjuvant Herceptin.

Once I completed my treatment I resumed what I believed to be a normal life style with simple changes, knowing I needed to make some dramatic changes over the coming months. Over the next 12 months I remained at the contemplating stage, having no answers, nor understanding the best way forward for my wellbeing.

Then in late 2014 my thoughts of change coincided with the discovery that I had secondary cancer recurrent in the right breast. Shortly after this news, after further investigation of a CT scan, they identified a white dot 6 mm in length in the left lung; with the aid of a FDG – PET/CT scan they confirmed it was cancerous and linked to the primary source.

Back to two key players in my life, I have been blessed to have inherited two lovely stepsons who have played a large part in summer and winter holidays for the past 22 years. It is great to see how they now are able to influence me in what I do. Both are extremely caring and were by my side during my treatment. I will always cherish those moments with fondness and happiness. It is a credit to them how they have supported Peter during my treatment.

With this new found knowledge I absolutely knew it was right for me to gain a better understanding of myself and my wellbeing. I elected to go down two paths of treatment and care, one under the care of The Royal Marsden the other looking at my wellbeing and life style choices with an alternative approach.

Amazingly I was introduced to Andrew Hunter in late October 2014 via a dear friend. He subsequently sent me a document, which I have explained in more depth in the coming pages. He knew from his own experiences that I needed to control my sugars and funguses intake into my body. These two items he believed to be feeding the cancer at the time. I set about following his recommendations to the letter.

In the January of 2015 I was under the magical hands of Mr Simon Jordon, a Consultant in Thoracic Surgery at The Royal Brompton Hospital London, who removed the white dot from my lung; this procedure is called bronchoscopy and left VATS single port apical lower segmentectomy. On awaking I was given the great news that it was a singular dot and he had successfully removed it, explaining it was only necessary to remove 10% of my left lung. In recovery I spent a few days in high dependency, a week on the ward and had a home carer for the following 6 weeks.

Treatment was ongoing and 6 weeks later I commenced 4 cycles of docetaxel/cyclophosphamide chemotherapy.

After my first round of chemotherapy treatment in 2012, I felt I was coping really well with this second round in 2015. My life style approach that included diet and care programme was working. I was only hospitalised once, with a low immune system.

After many tests it was agreed I was in good shape in June to have a mastectomy performed by the fair hands of Miss Nicola Roche, Consultant Breast Surgeon, in conjunction with a DIEP breast reconstruction under the care of Mr Paul Harris, Plastic Surgeon. Throughout all this time I was under the guidance of Dr A Ring, the Royal Marsden Oncologist, who managed my body with the right medication.

I was much more equipped at managing my recovery after these second and third operations and I put this down to many factors. Nearly 4 years on, from the start of the treatment it is still a bit of balancing act, but I feel in much greater shape than before. I would like to explain in the coming pages how I went about making these changes.

In writing this I have seen the pitfalls of modern life. Let me quantify what I am saying. There is no one to blame, it is all about getting the balance right to live in today's modern world.

I hope you enjoy my experience.

Prologue

In November 2014 I made a promise. "To look after myself to my best ability," this coincided with the news of having secondary breast cancer.

At the time I had no idea and in a state of fear and uncertainty, I set about finding new choices in my life. One thing I did know for sure was what happened in the past was not the right path now. Contrary to my belief the type and amount of sugars I ate daily from an early age were not giving me energy, but zapping my energy. With no blame, at the time I reached out for new ways for my life choices that would work in harmony with medicine and include the alternative approach.

In doing this I connected for the first time, to hear and receive sound guidance and direction.

The intention of this book is to show how no stone was left unturned, to inform cancer-sufferers and survivors and those facing critical illnesses you can improve your quality of life when you think your chips are down. You are scared and feel alone, you are not. Join me in the coming pages to show how with the support of many individuals I achieved something I thought impossible, being in perfect health. Equally this book is for anyone who wants to take responsibility for their health. Follow my story to see how I achieve this, by listening to my body, taking the right steps and feeling the benefits, it is incredible.

Interestingly as I explored deeper within my thoughts, I unlocked how dyslexia controlled my life choices for the wrong reasons. I discovered how I taught myself ways to survive within this cruel world as a youngster growing up, and remained in this attitude for far too long. It is my intention to share with you that you are not alone. You are as worthy as others. You are equal. You do have a voice and you can have a great purpose in life with a few key beliefs. I opened my heart, invited help and valued my own knowledge, it is with heartfelt gratitude.

Why was I inspired to write this book knowing my challenges with the English language?

My reasoning was the compelling belief that my message far outweighed my shortfalls.

The book is a testament to how hard things can be made simple and achieved with the right people's involvement, support, dedication encouragement and love during these past few years of turmoil.

I am sitting happy with the knowledge I have today. I am in the best place, balanced, calm and focused, nearly 12 months after my last operation. I remember the words of my Oncologist, 'you are unique. Yes you are free of cancer.' Those were incredibly comforting words to the ears.

I know this was achieved by everyone who helped me, not one stone was left unturned. There are many individuals behind the scenes whose roles or involvement played a critical part in my wellbeing, to whom I am indebted.

Throughout the coming pages you will see how distraction was the first brick wall I removed. I recognised the valve of how seeing the positives and negatives sit in the same place and can be fun to work with. I was able to realise even super-woman gets tired and needs to rest to prevent fatigue. These discoveries equipped me to explain my story during treatment of cancer without getting tired, a nice place to be.

Today I feel happiness in everything I do, life for me is rewarding and fulfilling. I find these new qualities give me time to do things with ease and confidence. I value my actions immensely.

I gained some insight into my life style that showed me that with the right mindset I could shift my train of thought and value my self-worth by being there to listen, not needing to be opinionated or solve the Worlds problems single handed, it is time to let others do so instead.

I cherish this knowledge. I have found "my life purpose" in sharing this with you.

The book style I have created allows you two ways to read it, first I suggest you read it all, and then later dip in and out for reference. During my recovery I made a promise to myself "to look after myself to my best ability". My wish is that you take notice too of my experiences.

With that in mind, you might be interested in reading further? If you hear yourself saying "that sounds like me," then ask yourself a few simple questions.

Where am I at?

What shifts can I make?

What differences can I create?

How do I feel?

Do I have that feeling I am missing something?
(That is not missing a bus, a friend, or a party, it is
deeper than that. This is coming from within)

What am I not hearing or listening to?

This book is not solely about my experiences during the treatment of cancer and recovering, but what it has brought to light is that there are different choices in life. I hope this equips you to consider your choices in the future?

Happy reading heartfelt thank you.

Contents

Time line   7

About the Author Sue Bannister   11

Prologue   19

Chapter 1:
Things happen for a reason   25

Chapter 2:
Open my ears to learning   33

Chapter 3:
How exhausting it was to tell others about my
secondary cancer at the time   41

Chapter 4:
Let others have their voice and
opinions without unbalancing me   46

Chapter 5:
Remove guilt and anger   53

Chapter 6:
Distractions are excuses   63

Chapter 7:
Creating energy helps the recovery   70

Chapter 8:
Scared is an acceptable state, I have learnt to
share my thoughts   76

Chapter 9:
Understand the value of positive and negative and
how negatives can turn into positives   86

Chapter 10:
Managing the mouth   96

Chapter 11:
Changing my eating habits   105

Chapter 12:
Pain control, living and managing it   117

Chapter 13:
Sleeping pattern change during treatment   128

Chapter 14:
The benefits of outside exercise   133

Chapter 15:
Recognising the difference in fatigue or tiredness 164

Chapter 16:
Say no with ease   177

Chapter 17:
Seeing the benefits of saying thank you
and feeling blessed   182

Chapter 18: Realise, accept help   187

Special note of thanks   197

Appendixes   208

Chapter 1:
Things happen for a reason

"It is nothing to do with good or bad, it happened for a purpose, accept what is!"

Yes it is what it is. I am still learning to let it go, move on and be thankful for that part of the past, With that in mind this is easier said than done, I know. I heard myself saying "why me" in the past for too long, thinking I must have been really bad for this is to be happening to me. You may be asking what changed my thought process? Difficult to recall, could I pin it down to one thing only? Maybe, there are lots of little and large reasons, but I would like to share how I moved from one thought process to a new one, to accept things in the past happened for a reason and I am the person who is best equipped now to deal with what is ahead.

Questions
Where do I start with this one, to accept?

Let me begin by setting the scene. Going way back to when I was bullied at school and singled out, I recall my Mummy always said to me, "if someone is talking about you, then there must be something interesting about you." So I accepted her reasoning and walked away with a smile each time someone talked about me. I learnt to adopt this approach to survive and accept I was different. Did I? No, not always, there were times I walked away alone and very hurt.

In 1973 the singling out by classmates at Portchester Secondary Modern was a breeze compared to the convent where I had been singled out far worst by the teachers. I learnt to accept I was best equipped to deal with what was ahead. I was treated as if I was different to my fellow classmates, I was allowed to do things others were not. This frequently caused unrest in the playground or after school. I had two choices, to accept I was different, or follow what they did. So it was my choice that I accepted the consequences, believing this lonely path at the time was right for me to survive my school years.

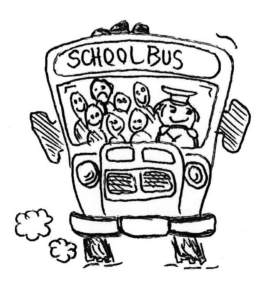

What made me feel good, when I was younger? My own freedom, cycling. Coming from a family with 2 elder sisters, it was a blessing getting outside in the fresh air. Too young to drive, it was my choice to cycle daily to and from Portchester to Hayling Island, a place where I started to forge life-long sailing friends, where I played on the beach and splashed about in the water, having lots of fun. During my long cycles I daydreamed of becoming a cycle racer in a team at one of those velodromes.

PROBLEMS AND MINDSET

The way I approached things as a younger to survive

I accepted I was different

Yes, it took me to a state of loneliness

This backlash hurt me when people talked about me

The belief this was the only option I had

I considered the time out on the bike in mid 1970 was helping me stay fit, so went back to the bike in readiness for the winter ski season. I knew the ideal training ground for this activity was tackling the steepest terrain I could find. Hill Road in Portchester was at the end of my road, not on the same scale as Sir Bradley Wiggins' training ground but enough for me. If I didn't make it to the top of the hill I went down and tried again until I did make it to the top. Little did I know then, that 35 years later in 2009, my childhood cycle training prepared me to cope with the cycle from Inverness to Petersfield in the depths of winter. The driving rain battering down freezing my legs on the Loch on the first day, coupled with a snow storm and whiteout conditions high up on the solitary road of the Glen as I approached my night's destination, Kings House Hotel just in time on day 2. (Before heading up the Glen I drew on my past experiences, calculating that even with the deteriorating weather I had the right experience and clothing for the conditions. Feeling confident that I would be fine to make it to the top cycling my bike, or at worst I knew I had enough energy to walk the remaining distance pushing my cycle in the thickening snow to the hotel). It never came to that, but 10 minutes after I arrived the road was closed for 12 hours, boy it was windy and the snow was deep. The scary thing was the hotel was the only building for miles up on the Glen, in total isolation.

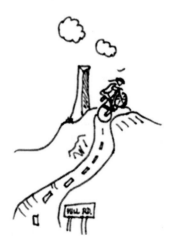

Thinking back yes I can see things happen for a reason, it all fitted in. OK I was disappointed I had failed my dream of becoming an international racer. Maybe as I didn't share my dream it could not manifest into reality, we'll never know. However, I believe I learnt very early that what I did in the past is for a reason, even with uncertainty initially, but how exciting it was when I knew I could cope with what was thrown at me the day up on the glen. So I had that underlying feeling I could cope with what was ahead now.

Have I answered this question? No not fully, I need to read it again. I accepted very early on in my life that things happen for a reason. But why me I don't fully know or understand. On a sunny September morning back in 2012 whilst walking the beach at Hayling yes, in my blue dress, funny I have it on now, I contemplated my thoughts. I knew I looked fit, every part of my mind body and soul was telling me something else. I had just completed working for The Corporation of Trinity House looking after the Austrian Olympic and Paralympics National House for the summer. I remember it was the week before I was told that I had cancer for the first time, (deep down I knew something was wrong, but I didn't know what at the time. I headed out walking alone on the beach at Hayling Island, I wanted to reflect and collect my thoughts, I knew I had loved everything I had done and felt complete and blessed. I know I was in the best place in my life, I felt calm still not fully accepting what life was going to throw at me in the coming months or years.

It is impossible to fully answer this question. My turning point though was shortly after reading a document sent as a gift by Andrew Hunter to me, his words resonated, I will explain more later on, this was just after I was diagnosed with the second bout of cancer. He taught, no he pointed out and explained by means of a document, that if I recognised that what was in the past was neither right nor wrong, life could feel lighter. It was my choice to move on. It felt right at the time. What he said made sense. I had to remember my thoughts of being on the bike and accept these things happen for a reason and I was in the best place now to deal with whatever was ahead.

What was the first process I had to take on board to deal with what was ahead?

The simple process of changing my breathing helped, along with letting go of the tension in my shoulders.

During the first couple of months I learnt to breathe properly by inhaling deeply. This helped and took away my anxiety. Let me explain. Sometimes when I am working or resting I would tend to take shallow breathes. Shallow breathing constantly is not healthy. When I continue to do it on a daily basis over a cumulative period of time it stops the natural flow of oxygen to all parts of my body, starving vital fresh oxygen which energises the blood to flow which gives me goodness. There was more than one technique that help me focus on breathing. In doing this it helped me gain a sense of calmness. I also took up meditation again, to help with these breathing techniques and deepen the level of oxygen entering my blood stream.

With this change I recognised it was my choice to accept that life has thrown things good or bad at me for a reason. It all had a purpose and in understanding those thoughts without the same level of worry I began to comprehend and view these experiences as magical moments of insight instead of apprehension.

What happened when I made the changes?

I felt calmer

I felt balanced

I can think more logically

I am going to ask myself, am I a better person? Let's think about that. I am surprisingly more comfortable with myself but it has not changed my character, nor have I put a mask on. If anything, it has taken down a veil.

It is a magical feeling this is the best way to describe my state. My body glows and radiates positive energy. It is natural for me to feel in a happier state of mind, my heart feels incredibly warmer and open. I welcome the place I am in rather than look at the negative points.

Am I a better person?

Yes I am calmer and balanced

Much happier state of mind

Life choices felt easier

I thoroughly enjoy that sense of freedom the bike brought me. It gave me time to reflect and happily take onboard what life has thrown at me. I am now at the place where I would like to explore what other options I have to consider.

Chapter 2:
Open my ears to learning

"What is open, if I listen am I open? No. So if I could learn? No."

Throughout my life I been influenced by my parents and siblings. Their thoughts and ideas served me in the family environment. As I grew up I wanted tó stand on my own two feet, show I was worthy of my purpose, and felt it was time to lead and take control of my destiny, not recognising it was strong to ask, seek assistance. I thought it showed weakness. What I wasn't equipped for was if I opened my ears to channel in and receive help and advice what amazing things could happen from it. When I opened my ears to listen and learn, I was astonished at the big shift changer for me. I am still really grateful and surprised by the abundance of support and help I continue to receive daily. Boy, it is a magical experience and I would like to share this with you.

Question
Why and when did I take stock of this initially, of not being open to listen?

Well it all started as far back as 1994 when I first went out with Peter. On our date I took us on a 6 mile walk. I learnt if you walk it is easier to listen and talk without distractions, and for those who know me I do get distracted easily and fail to listen in the process.

Over the past 22 years I have been with Peter, my dear husband. In my eyes I could never really grasp how and why he put up with some of my antics for so long, but he did, aren't I the lucky one! They say "love is blind" or actually really for me love is something that allows me to grow a special bond with Peter in my life. I feel blessed. Side tracked, distracted, going back to my tale of walking and why it works for me. I feel relaxed and free when I walk. When Peter and I have a difference of opinion and like to have good day out we don our walking boots and head outside for the beach or the hills. I normally come back nicely refreshed and in a calmer state after a walk with Peter. Our wedding anniversary was one prime example which started with a walk. (We walked half the length of Hayling Island, took the ferry cross to Eastney side of Portsmouth walked another 6 miles to take a surprise lunch at Royal Albert Yacht Club and walked back to the ferry, it was a magical day. A stiff breeze was blowing and we chatted and talked and I felt really alive that day). Peter had my attention all day, such a special day.

In the work place it came to me when I was working with Jessica McGregor-Johnson and Beatrice Buchser on Jessica's book launch. Beatrice was my buddy in the KPI 6 programme in 2011/12 and Jessica subsequently joined the team as an honorary member. On reading some of Jessica's book, things started to resonate that I didn't really have open ears, what I did have was selective hearing. I am sure I will not be the first or the last person to own up to going though life like this, and that things were not going to plan.

So here I am seeing a pattern forming with both Peter, and later understanding Jessica and Beatrice better. When I was with these individuals I felt relaxed with my train of thought. It was simple, there were no outside pressures, I could be myself. I happily opened my ears to listen to them, neither of them had any hidden agendas.

I suppose if I am honest and look deeper into the reason why I didn't listen beforehand, when I was at school it was because I spent all of the time in a state of fear. You may be wondering why? I was scared, thoughts like what was the point of trying to read out loud as I would stumble on words I could not say or understand them. If was really difficult to know where to start to pronounce the word let alone know what it meant. The sheer thought during those times spent in lessons when the teacher was asking one of us to read out aloud in the class, sent me into blind state of panic. As a little girl I sat there frozen rigid to the chair, frightened, stomach in turmoil, head/ears full of wrong ideas. So with that thought I never believed I had the capability to hold on to or learn anything, so why bother to waste my time in listening in the first place? I spent most of the time in a daydream hoping to shut out the panic and turmoil.

I hated those wasted days, always wishing I could be like a normal child. This could be why I closed my ears, (notice another excuse), or the cause of my reasoning not to open my ears.

PROBLEMS AND MINDSET

Recognising what took me to this state

Thought asking for help was a weakness

Caused me to be alone for too long

How did I feel making this shift?

The first big shift for me was when I was told the news that I had recurrence of cancer tissue in my right breast in November 2014, followed quickly afterwards by the news that they found a small shaded white dot in my left lung. After the scan my care treatment needed to change. I sat there numb initially, accepting the news. OK, absolute panic set in, I needed to think about this. Peter was really supportive, far stronger than I thought he would be. Our plans and priorities had to change now. How?

Let me explain, during my first diagnosis up to 2014 I would happily follow instructions from the experts to the letter to get to the right outcome. At the time I could hear myself saying it is not my field of expertise nor did I have the capability to understand the best actions if told what was going on. In those situations everything said rarely sank in, leaving my destiny in others' hands. In my train of thought now this wasn't a comfortable place to be any more but I still didn't know how to change this way of thinking. Until October 2014 I would allow and accept it was OK to let others take control of my health, now I asked myself why? This wasn't good enough now, I wanted to feel empowered of my wellbeing. My school years daydreaming had kept me too detached of any input and involvement in the outcome for far too long, other than being there in person. I had to change.

Even though it was my choice to make the shift, I still failed to know what personally I should do. Was it possible to change my thought process and did I have the capability to open my ears to hear as well as open my mind to learn what were the right steps forward for me now?

This is how I went about the change at first. This was the only way I knew how, to stand alert. If someone was talking to me I would check if I was listening, by asking myself subconsciously, "if I was listening?" If not, I would stop what I was thinking or doing, then ask them to recap, start again and repeat what they just said, apologising saying "I wasn't listening beforehand." This worked. The other fundamental shift changer for me was, could I made sense of what they were saying? Then having the ability to take myself totally out of the third person was unusually rewarding, now in the present state it was a weird feeling. When I didn't understand I asked them to explain in more detail. It was amazing what I was capable of learning and recalling. I do feel surprised and pleased with their reaction and my ability to take it all in. I am encouraged with the outcomes so far.

Remembering how I had made a promise yes to myself, it was my choice to seek the best way to look after my wellbeing to get me to perfect health. Still uncertain, I knew I could not achieve this outcome on my own, so I went in search of more answers and help.

My uncertainty brings me to a story or a bit of advice shared by a business mentor at a breakfast meeting, and I would like to share it with you. He said "to create something strong you cannot do it on your own." He told me the story of the Rothschild family, "how one of the Rothschild family was alone and went and demonstrated if you have one arrow and you try to break it in half you can do it easily, but if you have collection of arrows then tie them together in the middle, then try to break them, it is impossible. So with this in mind, this is how the Rothschild family modelled their business, without any money at the time, to create a bank, the unity of the family involvement built an empire, they are believed to be the wealthiest *family* in history." Therefore I realised, years later, that if I want to really succeed in life I had first better adopt their methodology in the practices of collaboration with others, build a team and partner with the right support to help me, first during my treatment, then again as I grow my business in the coming years.

What did I do next?

With this thought in mind the next thing I did was to reach out for support and guidance to help me open my ears to learn new techniques. Things came flooding to me, friends linked me to specialists then consultants put me in touch with the top specialist in their fields. How blessed I felt, I bubbling with excitement for the first time in years receiving and hearing properly, rather than selective hearing syndrome.

I listened carefully, I read everything thoroughly and asked questions, seeking guidance from specialists in their fields to explain when unsure, and trusted their advice.

What was it like having lots of extra help?

The most noticeable thing was, I was able to relax, learn, listen and question without any inhibition. It was a refreshing feeling. I see I have been using words like this a bit too frequently; who cares? Happy to shout out my great news, after all it is my journey and my choice in sharing this with you, a big eye opener honestly. I never realised how much fun I could have with help.

Question without an inhibition

Seeking guidance

And listen differently

Trusting others

With this new found understanding, what was the next step I had to face? The telling everyone about the recurrence of the cancer in November 2014.

Chapter 3:
How exhausting it was to tell others about my secondary cancer at the time

"Yes it was exhausting initially especially when I mentioned that the cancer returned, their faces told all"

What was alarming was how I initially reacted to their facial expressions, saying things like, don't start banging the nails in the box, I am not going anywhere. I explained the plan, at the beginning I was putting on a brave face, remembering at that time I was truly unsure of the outcome, indeed it was mentally and physically exhausting when I explained my situation. With time I was pleased to say once I felt I understood the pitfalls and outcomes I became calmer. I think this showed in my voice, actions and in my facial expressions, that I was happy to share my fears with friends who asked.

Questions
I had a lot of uncertainly which was exhausting in the first instance, why did it make me feel like this?

For me to explain that I had secondary cancer was a bit like trying to put pen to paper or having a tooth pulled, a painful slow exercise best avoided when possible. For those who don't know me it has been very difficult for me to formulate words on to paper. Here is an example; for years, this is how I would seek an alternative way to spell a word. It wasn't unusual for me to not know how to spell the first or second letter of a word. Finding the actual word in the dictionary was pretty much impossible. In those instances I would look at another word that I thought meant the same that I could spell, hoping that the similar word meant the same, at that point hoping the word I wanted to use was in the explanation. This was a lot of time and effort just to use a word.

Definitely a roundabout way, but the only way I knew, and at the time indeed exhausting. I still use this technique today.

In another around about way I believed that I knew what friends and colleagues wanted to hear about my cancer. It was my choice to come across at the time sounding confident with a plan. In trying to formulate this plan, especially with so much uncertainly at the time, I found whatever I wanted to say or write was for some reason being blocked from coming out. In order for it to come out less confused and muddled, I rehearsed what I was going to say. Somehow this did not sit right, but in doing this exercise it did come out easier. In my eyes I wasn't being true to myself, masking my true feelings and not speaking directly from my heart, consequently all these thoughts going round and round in my head were draining me physically and emotionally.

Whilst this was all going on, the conversation of cancer was controlling mine and Peter's life. He was equally tired and frustrated, quite rightly so, he had every right to feel like this. He was fed up when friends always asked about me. What about how Peter felt, no one ever asked, shame. Hence the backlash for a while wishing to change the subject or on occasions he would say "ask her yourself."

Was I right to be so flippant?

Yes and no. It isn't that simple. I know from my own experience that when I have heard someone say they have cancer I automatically had the worst thoughts. I know that sounds harsh or strange coming from me, that is the case, little has changed without knowing the whole facts. So little is known still about survival rates from cancer that it is worth sharing what I know.

Going back to my thoughts, my reasoning for being flippant stemmed back from my uncertainty or lack of understanding of what was going on in their heads and was potentially triggered because of my fears, or the shock of the expression. I didn't know what to really say next to reassure them. It was far easier to turn the conversation around. This was the only way I knew how to react. I felt deep down I would have thought like them in the past. Why it was my choice to be flippant was to put them at ease. Making light of the situation with my facial expression in the end was actually fun and we normally ended up having a bit of a laugh.

On reflection, after my fathers' first bout of cancer was diagnosed he went on to live happily for another 24 years with secondary cancer, though his cancer was caused by being exposed to fibreglass and asbestos, known as asbestosis. You would think I would think differently what to expect but I don't, or didn't at the time.

How did I turn this around so I was not exhausted?

I gained a better understanding of what was going on when I talked to others about my cancer at the time. There were a lot of things that contributed to me not being exhausted it began when I sought independent help, from different sources to talk more openly, for me this created the biggest shift physically and mentally.

One of my first wins was when I realised it was time to stop and listen to my body rather than trying to keep proving I could do it all. This was a great shift, as I definitely couldn't. One step at a time, I have learnt to accept help and to allow others to do things for me. The fundamental change was the importance of giving myself quiet time when tired or unsure, just to give my body and mind quietness.

I felt the need to keep my well wishers aware. This was time consuming and sapping me of my energy, so I looked at different ways that could still be personal. The most effective and simplest way of updating everyone seemed to be by means of blogging. The process of doing the blogs in turn helped me express my real feelings and give everyone a better insight of what was going on inside my mind as well as physically to my body. Doing this was therapeutic for me and took away the worries of many dear friends. A great benefit it cleared the ice when I next encountered them in person; our conversation was more fluid and more relaxed. I was amazed at the response of followers on the blogs alone; I would like to express my gratitude to you all from the bottom of my heart. Your support gave me inspiration and lifted me immensely during those days of uncertainty.

It was my choice and I appreciated the benefits of making these little changes. They helped me to stay balanced, relaxed and anchored, thank you.

What one lesson did I learn from my new actions?

How communities of friends are up-lifting. Thank you, you gave me courage and helped me remain positive.

Sought independent help

Gave my body and mind quietness

Helped to express my real feelings

I felt anchored and more balanced

A great way to start to aid my recovery, but what prevented me from moving forward with my promise I made to myself?

Chapter 4:
Let others have their voice and opinions without unbalancing me

"I have learnt how, when others voice opinions, to let it bounce off me, allowing them still to share their concerns and worries. This has given me a much greater calmness to handle what is ahead or around the corner."

For me now it is possible to remain calm and relaxed in the same state as before they shared their concerns, this is a big shift changer for me. My character over the years has not helped me, my excuse is I work in the service industry and my over caring nature. If someone in the past chose to share their woes with me, I would quickly take on their concerns and state of mind. This of course has been too heavy for me to carry onboard, totally un-balancing me emotionally. What I am learning to do, is still be there to listen, whilst reminding myself to think or say, "they are their/your concerns, not mine." It does not mean I don't care or listen, but by doing it this way I have learnt to let their inner emotions bounce off me, so this has allowed me to still have my own inner karma. Up to then I failed having a sense of calm. I actually found it almost impossible to have any inner karma. This was a dreadful state of mind to be in. I wasn't helping them or especially me. My plan is to show how I made the choice to make the shift as best as I can.

Questions
How did I contemplate shifting from one thought process to another in a balanced way?

I don't really know if it was one thing for sure, but I knew I could not continue down the path of 2012 that wasn't working. The first, then the second diagnosis of cancer in 2014 were the biggest wake-up calls I ever had. The medical hospital support was amazing. However, I was missing the point. There was something wrong with my inner balance. I was missing something, or is everyone else in the universe having the same experience? I don't know?

On reflection, November 2014 was a turning point for me, this was all new for me. Here I was sitting in a room in south London surrounded by ladies. It was a one day Instance Pause session being organised by Danielle Merchant. Her objective was to teach me tools to open up my thought process. This I understood was to allow me to look and seek new ways in life that would help me. An interesting thought, hence the reason I was there, hmm.

We started the morning off with personal introductions; I was extremely anxious, my heart was pounding as my turn loomed up. Spitting my introduction out quickly, I was relieved and ready to start the next task which was to create a graph to show my past 12 month highs and lows, the idea was to see if there were any insights from the patterns forming. Indeed there were, it was like a yoyo going up and down all over the year. All I could see was my whole world spiralling out of control, with my mother's illness, my treatment, the family, my pain. However, much I expected this and felt I already knew this pattern, at that moment of the morning I was baffled and uncertain of what this day was about and I felt somewhat frustrated doing this exercise. I believed she hadn't taught me anything I didn't know already. Or had she? Interesting thought, why had I paid her this money when I could have done this at home on my own, or could I? Hold that thought. (Appendix Instant Pause 2014 from January, and from July 2014 pages 209 to 210)

Alright back to the plot, that same afternoon I had to create a storyboard showing how I saw the next 12 months panning out in my eyes. When I draw it is a great way I can express myself freely and I normally come away relaxed. With no stones unturned, lots of ideas flowed freely and rapidly, the paper filled with colourful ideas whilst I created my amazing storyboard. I surprised myself how naturally it developed, especially with so much uncertainty happening in my life, the treatment that lay ahead or the outcome, this exercise gave me a great sense of calmness. Was it because it was my choice to create this or was it the fact I could look at ways I could feed and nourish my body and mind? It was magical to unleash and see new beginnings by creating this storyboard. This day's exercise made me understand it was time it was my choice. I could make this storyboard happen with care and attention, and the first step was showing me how to create a calmer year ahead. What was interesting, it gave me insights to explore how not to carry the weight of others' worries, which was another next big stepping stone to calmness, but how?

Now 3 years on I made this connection. Out of the blue I was introduced via Facebook to this human behavior and cognitive expert, speaker, educator and International author Tony J. Selimi. He came highly recommended and with nothing to lose I booked my first session with Tony in April 2015.

At our first session he asked me lots of questions. His questioning made me see that everything I was doing was not helping in my life. I had too many worries, many nothing to do with me, these were keeping me in an un-balanced state. This was definitely an eye opener for me, what an amazing session thank you Tony. I left his session feeling as if a big weight had been lifted off my shoulders. For the next couple of weeks I was in a much calmer, relaxed state of mind, wondering and having no idea what he had done to get me there.

PROBLEM AND MINDSET

I went in search of new ways in life that would
help me understand

Why I was missing the point

Insight to recognise that something was wrong
with my inner balance

Did it come easily making this shift to letting others have a voice?

For me to make the shift was surprisingly easier than I had expected. All I had to do was listen but not get involved, OK listen to me. Yes, I took the decision in April 2015 to remember that what was in the past wasn't going to change. I equally understood my character was not going to change either, hold that thought now. I recognised it was wise to change different aspects of my life but not my character, but I realised it was a good time to let others have their voice. With that in mind, and my belief that their concerns would not impact my feelings or emotions, I made headway, remembering to retain these thoughts as a prompt to remind me that if something did not serve me, to let it go, but remember to remain in the present to say "thank you" at the time.

OK on other occasions when I recognised my inner feelings were getting the better of me again, I had to remind myself to stop and listen and focus, remind myself that it is OK to be there whilst remaining distant and remember it is not my place to know how to solve the problems of the whole planet, nor does Sue always know the answers. With that thought, now I know it is the right time to let go of the ego aspect of my mind, I cannot always help. I was rather fascinated having this thought at first. Very interestingly it truly helped me in the early months of changing my thoughts, even during editing this still makes my stomach excited and wobble.

It was all new ground for me to tread, yes easier than I expected.

Explain how the inner calmness sits and the benefits?

I found it pleasing to have this inner calm. This is new, few situations at present unsettle me. Whether it be addressing an Ambassador or pulling together a team of volunteers for the first time, in both situations I feel more at ease and equipped to manage what my nerves throw at me. It is bizarre, I can now look over a balcony that looks down over a steep height with no fear. OK, my character is not an out-and-out worrier, but I am known at work for doing things right. When a client is nervous, that normally puts extra pressure on me which would have unnerved me. However, I have learnt not to show it. The difference now is that I am starting to feel more comfortable, it is a refreshing experience and I feel calmer than I have been for a very long time. I know this unrest creeps in now and again when I am tired, I look for tell tale signs and stop what I am doing, to rest.

Equally I have benefited from a new found ability to have a clearer mind with this inner calmness which is interesting; I have capacity to let new stuff sink in properly, to my surprise. Another thing I benefit from is being included more in conversations rather than being left on the side lines. I feel this was achieved because I have taken the time to listen and let others have their voice whilst I become the observer rather than always the doer.

I discovered I could tackle things easier. In the process of hearing I was less confused when something was said to me. I noticed when I stopped offering advice my friends looked at me less vaguely. You know, that look as if you have said something as if you had just landed from outer space, yes that look.

For the first time, yes, all in all, it is becoming easier for me to understand and digest new things. This is a perfect result.

It great to feel inner calmness

Refreshing to have a clearer mind

New things sink in easier

Nice to be included

What were the other things in life I wanted to change, did I have to rethink what I was thinking and why? Let me consider what other excuses have I hidden behind?

Chapter 5:
Remove guilt and anger

"Holding the thought of why guilt, anger or worry, does not serve me"

None of those thoughts are going to change the situation for good. It was only when I accepted that these thoughts don't serve me that life became calmer inside for me, yes the tension in my muscles started to ease. I started to recognise and took notice when I was getting tense, so at that point I looked within to see what triggered this behaviour. How did I learn to understand or to get to where I am now? Let me explain in the best way I can, how I believe I did it.

Questions
Why did I feel guilt and anger in the first place?

I held anger for other people's actions, as much as mine, for too many years for lots of different reasons I didn't understand why. In many situations there were times when I would have been excluded or not invited to be involved. In those situations it came across that I was excluded as they believed, because I couldn't read and write properly, I wouldn't have anything valuable to contribute. That felt horrible. I was left out frequently and this caused me frustration and anger.

Then there were lots of lovely situations I had, but I would like to share just two examples of how I let the wave of guilt encompass me just because I didn't write thank you notes. Basically that was an impossible task for me to do. I couldn't write, in my minds-eye there was no way of saying thank you properly, for which I felt ashamed and guilty at the same time. All of this negativity send me into a downward spiral mentally.

Thinking back, here is how lucky I really was. Back in 1975 I was invited by an Italian hotelier to train and ski with a local ski team in Cesana Torinese. For the winter of 1976 I took up Gino's gift, which was incredibly kind. I had an amazing time skiing with the girls and most of the guests in the hotel during that season. The season ended abruptly due to news of my father's illness. I returned home straight away to be with the family. Do you know I never made contact again, hearing from afar from another ski friend of his last years he spent in Flaine. Imagine how I felt?

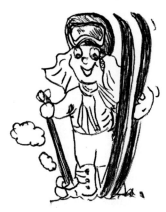

Now on home soil back in Hampshire, another lovely gesture. The Head of Portsmouth Historic Dockyard at the time, Commander Hart, arranged a ferry solely to take me to and from the Kings Stairs to Cowes main quay on the Friday of Cowes week in 1982, so I could watch the racing and visit friends sailing at Cowes. What an honour. What would normally happen is my father would be given daily passes to take the ferries laid on for the dockyard personnel and families during Cowes Week. However, that year the ferry service had been suspended due to the Falklands war. I was overwhelmed by the generosity shown. It was when I stepped onboard I saw this ferry was solely for me. What an incredible privilege, such an amazing gesture. And again I never said thank you in writing. Imagine holding those thoughts for so long, what they did to me? Over time my guilt manifested in anger.

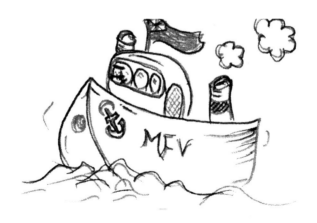

PROBLEM AND MINDSET

Ashamed of not making contact

I didn't think I had anything valuable to contribute

Felt excluded

Ashamed and guilty

Did I let go of the guilt and anger on my own?

No, not at all, there was a combination of factors that made me see reason. My business coach methodology was one of them, his introduction sowing the seeds on the opening morning of the 30 week accelerator pro-gramme. He said "what is in the past will not happen again, so let it go, move on." How true was he, this was a turning point for me back in 2011. Then again hearing how my buddy Beatrice and honorary buddy Jessica got together inspired me to let go. A few years later her Face-book page of Gratitude helped me realise how blessed I am with so many unique things happening to me in my life that I had taken for granted.

How did I become calmer and recognise that with guilt and anger came tension and what do I do to keep this in check?

With everything happening in my life since 2011 it was my choice to re think as recently as 2015 to identify what triggered the calmness within me. I looked at patterns. There were a couple of steps I had to adopt first, I had to accept whatever I did in the past could not be changed, I understood that from 2011. Guilt was not going to make the past any better.

The idea of using meditation for me to awaken myself to my body, was still relatively un-explored or used infrequently (on those rare occasions back in the late 70's I am surprised I only used meditation techniques to help me get through a busy Saturday working in the ski shop after a heavy night out on the tiles with friends). It was a really useful tool when I needed it. I am surprised now I didn't carry on to use it on a daily basis afterwards. I failed to realise the benefits until much more recently. Bearing in mind the practice of meditation was first recorded back in 1500 BC, it might be worth my while trying, since it has been tried and tested by millions in the East.

As recently as 2014 I was staying at Alexander House, south of Gatwick where I was with a girlfriend, Gillian, to celebrate her birthday. We booked ourselves onto a yoga lesson. At the beginning of the class I had to complete a form giving my medical history. It took me ages to complete the form. The instructor only allowed me to do the class with trepidation, considering I was still on a course of chemotherapy. I had selected the hotel because it was less than an hour from the hospital, so if I felt unwell I could get there quickly for treatments.

Anyway back to the plot, at the end of the Yoga session the instructor offered to send me a Yoganegra CD. As good as her word, it arrived in the post a few days later. She said it would help me retain and gain energy. I thought this was a great idea. This was a turning point for me. I was up for anything to help, remembering I wanted to give myself the best chance of wellbeing I practised it daily.

I soon benefitted every time I listened to the CD, a great tool. It put me quickly in a state of relax/calm during the months of my chemotherapy treatment and was a great anchor. The chemotherapy drugs were harsh, possibly an understatement to say the least. I got a lot of amusement practicing the Yoga at Hayling with friends they normally were snoozing a few minutes in to the session.

When I felt sorry for myself I would listen to the Yoganegra CD, or imagine I was listening to the tape. Whilst I waited for hours in the A&E department to be admitted in 2014 and 15, I used meditation on those occasions when my Neurophils dropped below 1, that was not a good place to be. I was rather poorly with no immune system to protect my body from the elements, however my symptoms were difficult to describe. I felt a fraud in a lot of pain, I was scared, tired, tense and totally exhausted. If you have ever had flu, it was worse than that. The only way I could calm myself was practising this yoga, it was a great comfort. Back in 2011 before I practiced yoga feeling frighted and scared the team at the local hospital at Epsom put me in a private ward even though I was a national health patient saying "they knew I had a long road to go and they wanted to make me as comfortable as they could." Their kindness made me cry.

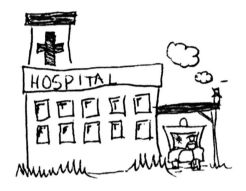

How crazy, could you believe it, once the chemotherapy had finished, I stopped using this Yoganega mantra? Strange, but I did. Duh, what was all that about? It is time to start using it again.

The second step in 2015 was to understand how to let go of the guilt and anger. Hmm that word again. I had to give some thought to that, I realised here at this point I needed a plan of action to move forward to keep me in a natural calm state of mind. This too would help me move away from the feelings of guilt, anger and tension. Easier said than done!

On reflection now, I forgot initially once I choose the path how easy the quick wins were. Knowing I enjoyed the habit of talking and walking, no walking and talking, for me it was relaxing to be chatting away. It was especially fun when I walked with a friend whilst taking in the fresh air, the miles seemed like a stroll in the park. Hayling beach provided a perfect backdrop. Thank you to Jayne, Sarah and Gillian.

Now it took another 16 months to really learn the benefits of practicing mediation on a daily basis. This wasn't until the April of 2015. I am a bit like my elder sister who is sceptical of the practice. What made me shift? I mention Tony quite a bit, I was having another session with him and commented I was annoyed with a situation with a client. I kept being challenged and it was making me nervous, I was starting to think I shouldn't be working with this client. I knew that what I was tasked to do, I could do with my eyes closed. But what I was hearing from the client was undermining my thoughts, which was annoying at the time. He taught me to let go of other peoples self doubts, they are not your doubts, you cannot change their state, but you can change yours, stay calm be yourself and all will be fine. I took a while to absorb what he had said.

I realised later I was annoyed and angry with the client's shenanigans and nothing I did would change them. Consequently this created a negative energy field around them which I didn't need to be part of. His guidance for me to think or say at the time was perfect, "I understand that is what you think, or it is your choice." Sometimes I would hold their arm and say, "yes that is how you think or believe it to be." A great release came to me doing it this way, I become calmer instantly. Without anger, thank you.

The other situation that caused unnecessary annoyance and anger was when Peter my hubby would say something uncharacteristic of his nice nature, by being hurtful in words. This was normally brought on or stemmed from out and out tiredness or frustration. What I did instead of being annoyed or angry or hurt, I shifted it to saying something like "that is not a nice thing to say," or that was rude, or that wasn't very loving." He normally was surprised at my response and would walk away, then come back later with an apology. The conversation stopped there and then, this action stopped a lot of negative energy being wasted, personally I see a much calmer state between us now. These three simple practices have made a big difference in the past months.

What were the benefits of this change when I believed I removed guilt and anger?

I was able to laugh more readily at things in the past that were normally annoying. I have learnt to stay neutral in situations when others were rude to me, leaving them to vent and letting them retain their emotions whilst I retained my inner calm. I recognise the past thoughts of guilt and anger were unnecessary, this freed up more time for me, allowing me to be in a calmer and more relaxed state.

Equally I recognised the world was made up of lots of different people and it was OK for not everyone to agree or always get on, when I came across someone like this I learnt to keep my distance. This was a more acceptable approach and worked for me.

It was strange how things flowed more easily, how changing my thought process has given me access to information I have accumulated over the years which I never realised I had retained. It was comforting and refreshing finding this knowledge flooding back into my head.

I have leant to embrace life. It is my choice and decision to see the world with excitement and passion, not with doubt or concerns. Remembering every wrong situation is an opportunity to learn and take stock of how to make the right choice in the future.

Looked at recognising any patterns

Accept whatever in the past will not change

Took to more walking and talking

Clear mind, freed up more time for me

I see the world with excitement and passion

My thought process does not reflect a defensive approach anymore, it is more balanced. I am happy to walk away, remembering those golden words. But what more can I do.

Chapter 6:
Distractions are excuses

"Excuses are reasons why I have remained in the same state for too long"

It is easy to confuse and combine being too busy with distractions; therefore I have made too many excuses why something didn't happen in the past. Yes, I fell foul of this state for too long, never having enough time is my excuse, rather than thinking what distractions are preventing me from doing what I want to do, and what I want to achieve from my actions in life. I heard myself saying I don't have the skills to write, rather than look at the benefits of what others will gain from me putting pen to paper and sharing my experiences. With this thought in mind I would like to share now how I came to understanding about distractions which then taught me to focus on my actions.

Questions
Can I give you an example of all my distractions?

Difficult to explain, here is on example. When I haven't yet finalised a plan in my head and thoughts are still floating around I very much remain in the creative stage, my head is awash with ideas. I am a visual person, lots of things stimulate me and consequently so do distractions. In the past my office desk 9 times out of 10 was awash with piles of papers, and I heard myself saying "well I know where everything is if I need something." I do stop periodically to tidy it.

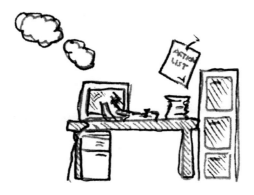

These days, I like to have a tidier office, but that doesn't always happen.

When it comes to doing things that make me tick, if I am not required to action it immediately I keep it out of mind's reach. I prioritise for later, with that knowledge it moves down the pile, that is my choice and style of work. In this state I naturally worked well to deadlines. I have always done it that way and I believe it works for me.

So here I am with an array of things mulling around in my head; may it be sailing at the weekend, how I approached the mark or how I sailed downwind, thinking about where we had our weight in the boat, what do I need to buy shopping, thinking of the list mentally; or I feel the warmth of the sun shining through the window and I consider if I should be going for a walk, or thoughts of my friend who's got a problem pop in, or I think it would be just nice to go for a coffee with a neighbour or contemplating if I should go and do all of the above; then my inbox just pinged so better have a quick look at what just came in. I know in the past my head was awash with all this, but I recognised that this needed to change.

Despite all the things going on above, I am still recognised for having plans and completing the plan on time. What happens having these distractions' is that I am constantly creating tighter deadlines, you know that is how I like it. I function better when it comes to events when the plan is pretty much formulated at the very beginning in work. I can visualise the whole event like a picture of many processes.

I believe my lifestyle prefers variety rather than routine, however, over the last four years I have taken lunch pretty much at the same time daily 12:22. Strangely given the choice I'll pretty much stop irrespective of what I am doing unless I am running an event or sailing.

There are two sides to my brain character both so different, one that is flighty, the other totally disciplined. When I am running an event I absolutely ignore distractions, it is amazing how I flip from one extreme to the other. PS haven't gone to lunch, it is the second side of my brain working now. With this consideration now, I know it is not healthy to skip lunch, so I stop. True to form it is 12:22 lunch time. I have to force myself to change my thought process to stop at times.

My husband gets really frustrated sometimes, but equally he has said in the past "he is amazed how committed and detailed I am when I need to get things done." Thanks Peter

How did I learn to recognise a distraction?

I first recall my early years from a school report my history teacher Mrs Wort wrote, "Susan is a lovely girl who is easily distracted, thank God she is doing geography instead of history." She was summing me up eloquently. It took me until years later; failing to listen nor taking notice of school, family members or my dear husband Peter. I bumbled along happily living with too many distractions, finding it impossible to concentrate on one thing at a time. I believed, in my work place this was great, it helped me keep on top of everything I did. Or did I.

PROBLEMS AND MINDSET

Excuses are when I am lacking focus

My head was awash with far too much

I found a way to cope and work to self created deadlines

What practise have I put in place to stop having distractions, or reduce them?

It took an outsider to make me realise my ways, I was having a session with Tony in May 2015 to pin down how I worked in my thought planning process. In my mind's eye up to then I believed it was my make-up, my DNA and nothing would change the way I thought. I was convinced that I would always be distracted easily, I believed I functioned better that way so kept making the same mistakes. He showed me some interesting techniques about me and my distractions and how to recognise why they happened; because I never put real focus on their importance I wasn't going to get rid of the distraction. With this new focus things changed.

Tony influenced me to do an exercise. Off I went and created a book of all the things I wanted to do over the next thirty nine years, starting with a time line from the start date to a finish date, setting out a budget, the tools or equipment I required to achieve each goal and setting out an action plan of the different stepping stones. It is strange, the book's gone missing, but I remember everything I wrote in it that I want to achieve.

In the book at the bottom of each page I wrote down "distractions will still happen but, I had to learn to recognise they are not necessary and prevent me from achieving my ultimate goals. Just let them go out off my mind and move on."

What benefits have come from setting my goals?

For once in my life, the fundamental difference is it is my choice to have this clear focus of my goals. Yes I can see them clearer in my mind's eye; they seem possible, achievable and real. Everything I set out to do with the right planning is comfortably achievable at the right time.

I have changed the way I think and waste less of my time in the state of wondering, and I don't hear myself saying "what if" or "if only" anymore, it is great.

Peter's response to the goals I select to share with him is amazing; he is so enthusiastic, his attitude has changed, on occasions he is more enthusiastic than me, which is lovely. It is much more fun looking forward with both of us working towards sharing these experiences and plans together.

When I share my goals with friends I feel blessed by their positive encouragement it definitely is incredibly rewarding and I am deeply touched by their support.

I look forward now with excitement to each day with new found energy and clarity.

Taught me to focus on my actions

Ability of seeing my goals are achievable

Touched by support of others

With that in mind what was my next step to help me on my way? Have I recognised that I am possibly doing too much, what should I do?

Chapter 7:
Creating energy helps the recovery

"I learnt how to aid my body into a much quicker state of good health by understanding the importance of keeping my own energy to myself"

I am known to have a lot of energy but what I failed to do in the past is keep enough for me, personally, at work. In sport I give everything away, giving my all, one hundred and ten percent. Well, that is not possible to achieve. With a big crash, bang and wallop I came crashing down at the end of 2012. What I would like to share now is how careful I am not to give all my energy away and the importance for me to retain a much higher percentage, not 50% but almost 100% during the recovery process to aid my recovery to good health. During this learning process I felt there were times of conflict as I had always focused on others rather than myself. This was sometimes hard to deal with. I noticed when others saw a shift in what they came to expect from me, this again caused me conflict. In the work environment it wasn't so difficult because I could delegate the task to a team member. In other aspects of my life I just had to learn not to get involved. I needed to let go, let others do it instead, it was now time for watching. Not a natural state of mind at first, but when I did, boy, the benefits were great.

Questions
What prevented me from keeping energy for myself?

During a session with Tony in September 2015 what he said made sense. The fact is it was my own self-worth holding me back from retaining my own energy. It is easy when someone from the outside explains, well I found it that way anyway. I could not keep my energy because I was doing too much. That is true to a point but not the root cause. Why, such a probing and burning question, why was I doing too much? It was my choice to do too much because I believed what I had done was not enough. This was my reasoning for wanting to contribute more, either in work or leisure time. I never stopped to think about importance of retaining some of my energy.

This is when I discovered a bit more about my own beliefs, my own lack of self esteem, call it what you may. My competitive edge was playing havoc with my mind. I always thought everyone or somebody else was better, taking me to a place where I thought it necessary to compete at everything. I wanted to be seen accomplished this is why I would happily take the lead all the time to keep proving I had self worth, how wrong was I? All I was doing was the opposite, falling short, missing promises I made because I was doing too much.

WAY FORWARD

Needed to recognise my self-worth

Others can take the lead

Meeting promises

Why did I have conflict when I decided to retain more energy for myself?

I never realised I had conflict about retaining my energy. I believed I was a normal individual like anyone else happy to give all their energy away daily. Well I know that is not actually true, those who hadn't contributed their all were in my mind's eye lazy. That is what I thought at the time. My circle of friends and colleagues were always keen to please and help, they say you meet like-minded individuals in life, maybe I did.

As I said earlier it just shows my naivety coming out once again. I thought the reason you went to sleep at night was to regain all the energy you used during the day. Therefore it was OK to use all my energy during the day in the first place as a nights sleep would allow me to replenish, waking up energised. I failed to realise that my lifestyle was far too active physically, and mentally my rest time wasn't enough, so when I woke up in the morning. I started slowly fumbling, around finding the simple tasks of making breakfast tiring. Could you imagine how I was going to get through the whole day? I didn't. I remember one day stopping the car, parking up on the side of the road for a good 20 minute nap, another time with nowhere else to go, I hid in a toilet and slept.

I never thought of this before, but all my constant activity was driven by self conflict. Little did I know, the reason I was trying to do everything was I didn't value my self-worth. Putting that aside, what I should have been doing was looking at what I could achieve with help; recognising just being present in some situations was good enough.

Faced with the reality check of wishing to be in a good state of wellbeing, it now became my choice to consider and take stock of everything I did or wanted to do. If I wanted to hold and retain and build my energy, something had to give, but I didn't like the idea of handing over the baton so I had to ask myself a few home truths.

A... I would ask myself in any action I was planning to do, do I want to use all my energy now, or shall I let someone else do it?

B... If I did any activity, what amount of energy mentally and physically would it take from me? Will it allow me to still hold some energy for myself, so at the end of the day. I would be in a position to be in a restful, calm state reflecting on the fun things of the day and able to unwind nicely ready for bed, rather than my body shaking with sheer exhaustion because I've done too much again.

This is still not easy, but I am getting better at evaluating what works best for my wellbeing in the long run. In October 2015, six months after my last surgery I still occasionally push the boundaries, and yes my body is quick to remind me to stop. My mouth goes first, or I lose energy like a flick of a switch. A harsh reminder when I have to nurse ulcers in my mouth. I am pleased to say they are getting less frequent. This is when I look at my nutrition intake carefully, which I have covered elsewhere in the book.

Do I really think I got healthier quicker by retaining my own energy?

Absolutely yes, there is no question about that. These are just a few of the things I did.

Once I grasped it was my choice to hold on to my energy I reaped the benefits; it enabled me to get better quicker. With this new knowledge, I found I could control my own destiny. I remember up to that point in time I was my own worst enemy. Things had to change.

I now happily sit quietly, relaxing, taking a sofa day, to conserve my energy and frequently tuck up in bed rather than watch a late film or disco at the Hayling Island Sailing Club. I understand I need to look after myself; the surgeon and consultants had done their stuff, but equally I had to make my choice to value the benefits of sleep when tired and rest when I felt weary. This is the key to creating a healthier me.

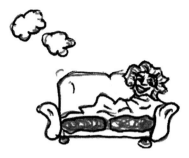

When I take stock and stop and recognise life is starting to get too busy I head to the haven of my Hayling house for a few days, to a far more relaxed setting having the comfort of the space, the quietness and the sound of the seas. The environment at Ashtead, sorry, is not a patch on Hayling. The time spent at Hayling allows me to recharge my batteries quicker, I always feel better from those few days. I come away refreshed and energised, time to head to Hayling Island.

Understand the benefits of retaining energy

Having the confidence to hand over the baton

Better control of my own destiny

Creating a healthier me

Happy to have a sofa day

Whilst all this is going on, during the turmoil what is going on in my head? Let me consider and explore this

Where was I sitting in my state of mind, did I understand the consequences of my thoughts?

Chapter 8:
Scared is an acceptable state, I have learnt to share my thoughts

"In my situation by not knowing the outcome in front of me, I was scared and thought I was heading out on this trail alone. This was so untrue, I shut out support of many, all I had to do was talk, there was always someone there to share my thoughts."

Life pressures and the uncertainty of illness made me scared, therefore placing automatically extra tension on every area of body, soul heart and mind. It is daunting, being in this stage of doubtfulness, it heightens the tension level in every muscle and has caused me to operate constantly in a state of shock, has created a rather hard place to live for long periods at a time. Once I understood how being scared affected my body, mind and soul. I knew this wasn't a good place to be and had to do something about it. Therefore, change had to come about, so I learnt it was acceptable to share my fear, I realised I wasn't on my own and I worked though this state by learning to release a lot of tension within by using different techniques.

Questions

What state was I in and what was going on?

I still believe I remained in this state, it could have been for two other reasons because my head was starved of nutrition and the worry over the years. Having a poor diet for too long pulled me down in a spiral; later on I have explored this in more depth. Then I think when the cancer took hold and got an anchor inside me, it changed how my mind, thought process and body functioned. (I don't have any scientific evidence but I am interested to know more if there is anyone out there who does have this data. Off on one of those distractions), OK not only was I tired, but in 2012 parts of my body hurt. If I knocked my right breast or if I lay on it was really uncomfortable, also I recall that the right armpit was tightening and painful to move. I was rather unsure of what was happening, opting for physiotherapy because at the time I thought all this was the effect of the menopause and stress. As I couldn't pinpoint the reason I was scared, plus I failed to ask the right people possibly made it worse.

Was I in a blinkered state for a reason up to then?

Briefly, for me having blinkers was the best way to cope at the time, my safety mechanism or whatever you like to call it. I was scared, for me this was the easiest way. I never explored any other way.

At the time I would have liked to have been in a situation where I could turn my reasons for being in a blinkered state on and off, like a light switch. I was sure this was not possible, this is what I believed. I could not have been so far from the truth. I didn't have to remain living in a blinkered environment. All I really had to do was make my choice to stop and breathe, to be open and to relax, to close out bad thoughts of being scared which created this lonely void, remembering I had the support of so many individuals.

Why did I think I was alone and scared, when I had so many loved ones, family friends and professionals around me?

Good one here, it stems back maybe because of my self-doubt. It is indeed a cruel place to be alone. How do I begin? When I found out for the second time I had cancer 2014, possibly on reflection this was the scariest time for me. The first time I generally could manage with what was ahead. No that is not true I was in a state of shock and yes I was scared in a different way of the unknown, my tummy was churning. The fear hit me more in 2012 during the rounds of chemotherapy treatment which caused me to end up hospitalised three times. The poison in the drugs was wiping out my immune system which should have protected me, this is known as neutropenic. Strange to say whilst in the haven of the hospital I felt safe.

How did I cope? Well I hung on every word I was told by the professionals. I had no reason to doubt them, they were very thorough and extremely helpful. What

I hadn't grasped was that there were others out there who could support me mentally as opposed to just the physical side of the treatment. I had learnt to shut everyone out in fear I would show how scared I really was, how could I change this thinking? To give you a bit of background, I was faced with reality check when I met my second consultant in 2014, Miss Nicola Roche from The Royal Marsden an amazing individual, so committed and kind in her approach. She believed that my tissue in my breast was at a pre cancerous stage and the cancerous tissues possibly in my lung were the same. Now, she said "as the horse had bolted they normally would monitor it, rather than operate." First she wanted to refer me to undergo some more tests with another consultant who specialised in the lung field. This referral took longer than I wished, but they were beavering away behind the scenes to sort it out for me.

The question concerning my consultant Miss Nicola Roche; was it linked to the original breast cancer and was it singular? Nothing was confirmed until they did a biopsy in late December 2015 at The Royal Marsden at Fulham. Still unsure, this was the first time I was petrified. Whilst they were doing the procedure of entering my lung using local anaesthetic going through my back, when they penetrated my lung I coughed. Unaware of the severity of the test, I had no idea they wanted to keep me overnight to check my lungs didn't collapse.

However, all the time I kept my thoughts to myself, trying to understand what was going on.

I see now my fear came from not sharing, thinking I might freak out my husband even more. He amazed me how he coped so well. During my first treatment Peter was by my side all the time. If anyone was alone it was him. He was incredible, didn't abandon me, no one did, I just felt like they had.

It was my choice also to keep my inner fears from my sisters and dear friends. I later shared much of how I felt, but possibly in writing this is the first time I have really shared my actual feelings. Yes on occasions I would have an outburst this normally started with welling up of tears, quietly sitting in the corner saying everything is too much for me. Up to now those moments were only shared with Peter and Sarah in New Zealand my oldest and dearest friends at Hayling Island.

Friends came from afar thank you Michelle from Sydney, Sue Parkin from Connecticut, Beatrice from Zurich and Jessica from Almunecar, coupled with always being there the visits whilst in hospital by Jayne, Sarah, Gillian, Richard and Simon, Claire taking me out to the garden centres and Melanie coming round with Bea was magic. I felt blessed and calmed when they were here, it took away the loneliness, my friends' presence lifted my spirits greatly. Even with the tonnes of well wishers cards and emails and facebook, I felt like I was facing this all alone well that is how I thought. They were always there with open ears but I still wanted to protect them. It was my choice to remain scared and alone for far too long without sharing my thoughts keeping everyone at arm length.

This was all enhanced because my network of dear friends were based at Hayling Island and I felt isolated spending all my time at Ashtead as I came under the treatment arm of what I believed to be the best hospital equipped to look after me, yes, The Royal Marsden Hospital in Sutton and Fulham.

Now under the care of Mr Simon Jordon at The Royal Brompton, everyone including me wanted to get to the bottom of this white spot in my lung, quickly. Just like magic my phone rang, whilst on the train home returning from seeing the consultant. He called to say they had a cancelation, which meant they could do the operation the next morning. It was now 4pm, oh, my gosh! It all happen so fast, get home, pack an overnight bag, called Peter giving him the news. Neither, Peter or I had time for it to sink in. We sneak in a quick dinner then he dropped me off, tucking me in for the night at the hospital. For me it wasn't until 10 minutes before going down to the theatre I felt scared. No time to share my fear. I was now in the fair hands of my surgeon.

Who was the first person I shared my fear with?

Honestly Sarah and Peter, I think it helped for two reasons, Sarah was a long way away coupled with the fact she had a gift of listening without being opinionated. Yes she is opinionated but in a different way, her compassion during my mother's death was incredible. I am so blessed to know her, she gave me insights, and was so kind in sharing her life skills in supporting me during my time of fear and uncertainty. She showed me ways of expressing myself, not to be afraid, to cry, to let go. She got me to see what was in the past was fine to let go, enjoy the happiness in doing what I am doing now, celebrate doing something for the last time with fun. Her compassion, helpfulness and calmness during my mother's illness and death in October 2014 was like a gift from heaven, she made things less scary.

So when it came to Sarah finding out I had cancer for the first and second time she didn't go into panic mode, she took time to listen and understand where I was at that moment myself. I cried with her on the phone and she was so caring, I cannot begin to express my gratitude, thank you Sarah dear friend. The doors opened, it made sense to share my thoughts with Peter my nearest and dearest so I did, and then my blogs came during the second round of treatment to my friends sharing the good news and what was happening.

How did I get out of this stage of mind?

It all started when I opened up, OK there is a big difference between talking and opening up. It was all about considering what was in my mind if I choose to share these thoughts, or just some of them. Sarah first then Tony in April 2015 gave me a release mechanism to see it from a relaxed state so that I could understand and accept what has happened and was going to happen will just be. What was in the past was in the past. What is in the future is the same for everyone. We all have choices, it was my choice, yes just like that, to change my thought process from scared to excited, both having the same meaning but from fear came a new found excitement, a fun way of approaching life changes. I accepted the unexpected, saw things differently and learnt to accept it from a different perspective. It may be an interesting opportunity, feeling blessed about what will happen next in my life.

Once I made the shift after 55 years into my life, I experienced a groundbreaking change in me and my outlook. It made sense. I didn't feel scared, I don't believe anything will make me scared again, because of my past experience, time will tell. Truly I do feel really blessed and grateful for this insight into how I came to change my thought process in my mind, yes it was my choice. Interesting that a one word shift from scared to excited made the difference.

WAY FORWARD

I opened up by sharing my inner thoughts

Looked through the same eyes differently

I didn't feel scared for the first time

What are the benefits now?

Ironically what was in the past seems of little or no significance which is great, so I find I am not fazed or scared these days, few things worry me.

My moments of unsettledness are less and less. I recognise I am only a human being and I see how perfect can be viewed in different ways with imperfections. This for me creates a calmer space within my body and mind. This is how it was my choice to understand the benefits of being in a relaxed state:

I learnt how to speak and open up and ask for help

I feel an abundance of support from friends who are eager and happy to help

I feel happy to be on my own and enjoy quiet space

The moments of hiding away from the real world have vanished, because I now have the ability to recharge myself with thoughts of tranquillity and meditation

It was refreshing and now fun

I have lots more happy moments I would like to share

Fear is a word that is created in the mind, and it is surprisingly easy to dissolve the fear to excitement

The past seems of little or no significance

I recognise imperfections are acceptable

I welcome an abundance of support and value their help

Life is full of excitement and happy moments

With this new found knowledge what next avenues will I explore to aid me in future life changes?

Chapter 9:
Understand the value of positive and negative and how negatives can turn into positives

"Once I understood that everything is counter balanced both ways in life, my life flowed with abundance of appreciation and gratitude, from this amazing things have come my way"

My mind was masked with thinking that you can only think positive, as negative thoughts were bad. So, for years off I went to read lots of happy, positive thinking books, thinking this was the right way forward but deep down, it didn't sit right. I felt I was missing something, as the positive energy within me was only temporary. Was I happy? No not really, not all the time. Consequently I never really considered until I was guided by my guru who showed me how to realise I could have as much fun with negative situations and thoughts, by seeing the positive in them. It is my objective to share my thought process now with you.

Question
Emotionally how did I feel before I understood that positive and negative both have a place in life?

My state of unrest and my emotional turmoil stems back to at least two years before being diagnosed with cancer. This state got worse when I was on my own. I felt lost and alone holding lots of doubts and negative thoughts. Don't get me wrong, I had lots of fun and happy moments with friends, but somehow they got lost and forgotten quickly when I was alone.

Let me share when I thought something was wrong. When I was in India, they say "a place of Sensation", how lucky was I to be invited on a formularisation trip of such grandeur. The journey started flying Jetindia business class, wow! During this whole trip we were accompanied by a private guides and this small party of 6 had a taste of living the high life, first in Mumbai staying in one of the finest hotels overlooking the bay, prior to a short flight up to Udipur for the second part of this trip were I was lavishly spoilt. Our second destination was like stepping into a James Bond film set, staying in the award winning Oberio Udaivilas, the most opulent resort hotel I have ever stayed in. Well actually it was more like a palace; I practised yoga in the stillness by the outside affinity pool in the early morning with the sounds of morning chorus. It was more than special, it was sensational.

You might ask where am I going with this story, ask me what I was thinking? Was I excited? Not at all, lost in negative thoughts, I found it difficult to join easily in conversations, nothing flowed, my brain was awash with pounding negative thoughts nothing could shake me out of it. Sensing it best to stay aloof it was my choice to remain quiet, remain detached from the team, God only knows why, we all came from similar interests but I didn't want to dampen the spirits of the rest of the group.

WAY FORWARD

How to get out of state of feeling lost and alone

Lost my excitement

Conversations didn't flow

On the last night, excited to get home possibly, or plied with lots of cocktails back in Mumbai sitting at the bar I shared my duck story with everyone, the whole party thought this hilariously funny and wanted to be part of the ducks tale. How the duck came to be with me in India, my hubby Peter has a really old small Snoopy toy which we always took him everywhere we travelled. However Snoopy is not mine to take, so I wasn't allowed to bring him, so as second best I took a little duck I brought Peter for valentines' day.

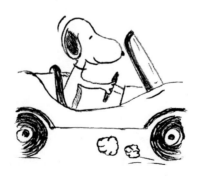

This was permitted, so I embraced the time with the duck as if he was my Snoopy. (Peter subsequently had a sneaky read of this and got most upset when he read this bit about Snoopy being described as a toy, "Snoopy a little person with feelings.") I have to agree with Peter.

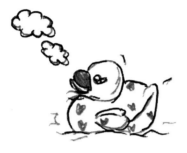

This was the first time I really engaged with them, we got up to some crazy fun things creating adventurous shoots where the duck paddled in the indoor stream at the hotel and popped him at pride of place at the front entrance of the hotel, where every time we were cleared through the heavy security system and greeted by the concierge on arrival. It was a hoot, I know I almost wet my pants with laughter, I saw the old me back having fun and I loved it.

In quick succession my work took me to Venice for another formalisation trip, this is one of my most favourite cities. Yet the same happened again, let me set the scene. I stepped-off the plane at St Marco airport to our host waiting to escort a few of us to the awaiting private launch to take us to The Cipiani The Belmond group flag ship hotel. Known for being frequented by the rich and famous and me, yes one of the finest hotels in Europe possibly the World, the trip was top notch.

The opulence continued with a return trip on the Simplon-Orient Express taking us from Venice to London. On boarding I was escorted to my private couchette by our porter, I got ready for my evening dining onboard whilst heading through the Austrian and Swiss Alps. I would best describe it as stepping into an Agatha Christie murder scene on the Orient Express unfortunately I would have been cast as the solemn dark character out to lure suspected guests that night. I did try with all my might, absolutely, dressing up in this sweeping long metallic dark blue dress with diamonties sewn on the front, hair rolled up make-up on, I looked stunning if I say it myself. Nothing, no thoughts of happiness would shift that solemn look or draw out a smile on my face. I remember entering the dining carriage hearing the piano playing as we took drinks before dinner, again I sat quietly. I think even if you had put 200 volts underneath me there was no chance I would have smiled. I found it really hard to engage in conversation, still with a head full of negative thoughts such as, why am I here? What can I do for Belmond Group, there is no chance I give them any business? Well those were stupid thoughts. I know that now.

With all this running around in my head it was exhausting, it was wearing me down. For those who know me I am the first one to be bursting with excitement, telling everyone about the magical experience and incredible opportunities and how India and Venice would work perfectly for the right company events, both very plausible options.

What I realised late, though it was shortly before being diagnosed with cancer, I couldn't express my true feeling, and hid at home rather than go out and do the things I loved doing. I would sit and watch TV, tidy the house, make excuses to remain inside. I shied away from crowds and good friends, beating myself up, totally miserable knowing I was missing out but didn't know how I could bring any enjoyment to the evening so remained away or only choose to go out in small groups. This was when I was at my lowest moments, I never realised this was possibly caused by the cancer, causing my thought process to keep me in this negative state at the time.

I lived to believe everything good was positive, and negative was a dark place to go, and never looked to see you could have as much fun with the negative side of things with a positive slant. Looking back I was in a desperate place to be only seeing myself spiralling downwards. I kept looking for answers or other ways out, but they didn't come.

How did I see sense and understand both sides?

It all happened really quickly, yes my state-of-mind shifted strangely when I got diagnosed, may it have been because I now knew something was causing me to be like this that it all made sense? I was definitely seeing the positive side, the support of some incredible individuals at the hospital, where I was pretty upbeat eighty percent of the time. It really only changed properly when I saw the pitfalls of my thoughts and behaviour feeding my positive and negative thoughts. When I was diagnosed for the second time, I realised how cancer had played a part in all of this, when reading Andrew's documents and Tony confirming what Andrew had stated.

I would say the biggest shift came when I recognised what Tony was pointing out, no, he didn't point it out, he got me thinking in a different way. He has a cunning way of getting me to realise it made sense this way, there are always two sides to things, some shapes have more, but we are talking about me and positive and negative thoughts they have only one side for each of them, but actually positive and negative have two sides. I like to describe the best way I can demonstrate my thought process. He helped me in this one session to become balanced, thank you and bless you Tony. OK, let me get back to the plot, in setting the scene, it has been raining all day, it is hot sunny day.

Look at the positives side for a rainy day

It will be good to enjoy a nice hot bath when I get back

I can appreciate a nice hot drink as it will warm me up from the inside out yummy

When it rains the High Street is nice a quiet and it allows me to concentrate in my own space when I walk

I can splash in the puddles what fun

Perfect weather for ducks

Look at the negatives for a sunny day

I get tired quicker in the heat of the sun, causing me to do things slower

I will get thirsty

Another thing to carry lugging this extra water around with me

I am in a hurry, the action of having to put sun cream on so I don't get burnt will cause me to be late, and it will hurt keeping me awake all night if I get burnt

I hate sun stroke, oh I wish it was raining

With this rational way of thinking he has shown me by writing down lot more examples how simple my mind works. I truly would say it is worth if you have time to checkout Tony J. Selimi or book a session with him, I found it worth spending this time with him.

What was the best thing that came from doing this exercise?

I learnt to appreciate is absolutely natural to have thoughts from both sides. For me the best thing was being more open with my positive and negative thoughts, but not to dwell on the negative thoughts or look specifically for them. I have learnt an easy process with the help of Tony to now take me into a positive state of thinking, by looking at the great things I can do when I turn the negative into positive situations. I feel I have reunited with my sense of humour, yippee.

Then there is the mind thing, when I hear myself saying that was a really big win, I have so much, absolutely am thankful for everything I have and do, I count my blessings more openly. It just took me longer to see the light and all the lovely things that are happening around me. I hear myself laughing more inwardly and outwardly. My vocal cords are relaxed, my voice doesn't go so deep or too high as frequently, that means I am calm and more balanced in my thought process. The signs I look out for if I am anxious or have negative thoughts, I know and hear the tone of voice change, funny I am conscious and now listen to it and say why? Reminding myself to stay relaxed, yes I feel I understand myself much better, I recognise I am here for a purpose and cherish every moment enjoy both experiences now with open arms.

I am more excited these days which is a lovely feeling and yes my voice does go sweaky but actually that is fun I like that character in me when I am excited rather than anxious, look how far I have got.

It is as easy as a flick of a switch

Seeing the positive side of negative view can be fun

Became more open and relaxed

What was the worst thing that came from this exercise?

I don't like to think too much about the worst now, as I feel I would be wasting my energy giving you all the negatives going back over old ground. My only lesson came potentially later than I possibly would have cared for not realising I could control this thought process much sooner that was my downfall.

My lack of self-belief was another one of my pitfalls that kept me in a state of denial of my own destiny. All the rest I would say are excuses not reasonable answers.

It been really rewarding challenging myself over the past 9 chapters. I've discovered so much about myself I had forgotten or never looked at closely before. The next stage is look at the way forward, where do I start?

Chapter 10:
Managing the mouth

"The mouth is the gateway to wellbeing, once I cherished its importance, I was rewarded"

Preceding cancer my mouth and tongue were never really right. Never did it dawn on me that all the bad bacteria forming in my mouth, caused by my lack of dental hygiene along with the poor diet as a child contributed to my mouth ulcers and potentially my wellbeing. At an early age I was plagued with ulcers and frequently suffered from a tender tongue, which caused lots of discomfort which regularly hurt me. Never at the time did I really grasp the essential reason behind it. My objective is to share with you how I began to understand the importance of how looking after the mouth would make such a fundamental difference to my health and wellbeing. This really didn't come to light until actually after my second round of chemotherapy in 2015 when reading the notes I kept. It is incredible it took that long, now I have continued to look out for changes during and post chemotherapy to remain healthier.

Questions
What I remember as a child?

After everything I have learnt, I think it is worth reflecting as a child the importance of cleaning one's teeth. At no time do I remember in the early 60's being taken into the bathroom as a child whilst in Portchester to be shown the right way to clean my teeth, nor even being checked, or watched over when I was cleaning my teeth. What I do remember was, at the dental surgery sitting there petrified, hearing the drill from in the isolation of the waiting room, frightened to the core, knowing once I stepped into the dentist's chair, it was going to hurt. I recall the dentist inflected pain every time I visited, by either an injection when penetrating deep into my gums or the moment he hit my nerve whilst drilling, even worse when he pulled out a perfectly healthy tooth. I was fair to say I loathed this experience. Therefore, I subsequently shied away from visiting the dentist for many decades. My lack of care caused a lot of bacteria to thrive in my mouth, this gave my ulcers a perfect breathing ground to survive.

How did I cope beforehand when my mouth was sore?

Honestly, not very well in the early years, I remember taking whatever was offered from my mother, Bongella, Strepsils, those usual products never worked. I found it difficult to talk, eat or drink when I had an ulcer. Riddled with pain I had many sleepless nights, and my mouth caused me many days off school and work. No thought was considered about why I was getting them in the first place.

How did I manage the problem?

Faced with this problem for years I soon learnt much later in 2014, it was better to stay off acidic drinks, sugar, tomatoes, salty crisps; the ulcers sent me on to a compulsory diet. There was a positive side to it, I believed. I discovered if I gargled with salty hot water the pain went away quicker. Back in 2011 when at my sister's house at Treeview did I hear how the bad bacteria stayed in my mouth when using an old tooth brush. She washed hers regularly with TCP, seemly it worked. Did you know it also helps get rid of common colds? She has an amazing white set of nashers; it was definitely worth listening to her. Thinking back, I don't recall she ever complained of having ulcers in the mouth either.

With a new lease of life in 2014, now rinsing my mouth out with salty water coupled with a clean tooth brush helped the ulcers go away quicker. What I didn't work out was how to stop them from coming in the first place? During the treatment the doctor prescribed me with hydrocortisone 2.5mg muco-adhesive buccal tablet. On top of this I would gargle with aspirin, always spitting it out. This helped bring down the swelling. Both seemed to help and worked well together.

WAY FORWARD

I asked my hygienist the best way to clean my teeth

Keep the mouth moist

Clean tooth brush

Talking with doctor

Who drew it to my attention that it was what I ate that caused it?

Hmm. Been using this word a lot, let me think, going back to when I was attempting to be fit after the first diagnosis of cancer to map out a life after recovering from treatment, I attended a talk organised by the team the Royal Marsden at Fulham start of 2014. In the audience were fellow survivors. Everyone was there for the same reason and we all listened, they asked us what goals we had and if we would like to share them, I did, (I wanted to compete in the nationals the summer of 2014 in the Flying Fifteen). They all agreed I could do it, (which I did). Back to the plot, in the reception area there were a few make-shift stands with booklets which explained that it was necessary to have a good balanced diet, not necessarily cutting anything totally out, just cutting back and doing things in moderation. I realised what they were saying was a good idea and I should be doing it, but their plans wouldn't work for me because I could not eat anything with dairy, that was my issue. So, OK, I knew what I was eating was not ideal, but what was I to do?

Sometime back Sarah Armstrong, my dear friend in New Zealand, called with advice. She gave me a whole list of things to eat, not to eat, books to read, what to do. She has been so kind and such a dear friend. I took notice by starting with lemon juice in the morning, and cut down my intake of coffee, removed decaf from my diet and went on to green tea. However what with the information coming from the hospital I couldn't filter all this information in at once. I was overwhelmed, it just didn't sink in totally and possibly I missed a lot about why my mouth was having all these ulcers, I was still unsure what to do.

Then there was Andrew's belief that my immune system was run down because all the toxins in my body were contributing to the mouth ulcers, like alcohol, refined sugar, caffeine, and lots more, I knew it was time to take stock and work out how to keep on top of this problem. I had to bear in mind, that Jane Dorey Chartered Physiotherapist, Grad Dip Phy MCSP, Stage 4 cervical cancer survivor, understood cancer at a cellular level, another source of great helpful information explained that most products we use daily have too many toxins in them. I had to change those too, to only use natural or raw products in everything I eat, drink or wash with was my first step. Indeed I threw a lot of things away in the coming weeks. *(see Jane's rough notes in appendix 208).*

What did I do that really made a difference?

At the very early stages of my treatment I kept a log. It was my way of keeping control of what was going on, by looking at the information I had logged, I worked out what triggered it during the first round of chemotherapy. I recognised once my tongue went, everything else went and consequently I would end up being admitted to hospital the worse for wear and remain there until I felt better. Surprisingly it coincided with my ulcers.

With recognising what triggered all the problems with my mouth, I could do something about it, so let me first explore what these were:

The poison from the chemotherapy treatment

Losing my appetite prevented me from having the right nutrition required for my body

I understand that being deficient of vitamin B12 was a key one

The treatment caused me to have dryness in the mouth

The mouth needs moisture to repair efficiently

Lack of sleep, the sheer exhaustion was sapping my energy

How did I manage to get rid of my ulcers:

I had a lot of medicine prescribed by the hospital my GP was great, giving me extra medicine to calm the mouth down quicker whilst I was having chemotherapy treatment

A gentle gel clear to wash my mouth 3 times a day to keep it moist, prescribed by The Royal Marsden

Drops designed to coat my tongue and take away the tenderness, this allowed me to eat

A hydrocortisone capsule I would suck under my tongue to reduce the swelling during chemotherapy treatment

My alternative natural herbs were not prescribed by the hospital or the GP but recommended by Jane Dorey who had secondary cancer herself similar to me:

Insode 3 carbinol 1 capsule a day (no longer available in the UK)

Milk thistle 1 capsule a day

Ubiquinol CoQ 10 - 100 mg x 3 a day

Health aid vitamin D3 1000 x 2 sprays a day

How to prevent and balance the mouth during treatment?

Drink lots more filtered water

Make sure I ate food which contained vitamins B12 such as meat, salmon or mackerel and eat lots of fresh vegetables

Listen to my body, stopping myself from doing too much, rest when tired

Change my toothpaste. Under the recommendation of Jane Dorey, I now use aloha and fennel or just aloha based products

Absolutely stay away from fluoride products

Keep my toothbrush clean wash it out with TCP or in boiling water regularly, thanks Catherine

Change my toothbrush twice yearly

Keep my gums and gaps between my teeth clean

Wash my mouth out with salt during the chemotherapy treatment, or when tender

Strangely, after noting the one above, cutting out eating salty foods, crisps etc.,

How do I make sure it remains in a good state?

This is a balancing act. I don't always get right as I have said before. After a spell of 5 days in Epsom hospital and slowly recovering, I requested a meeting with my Oncologist Dr Ring at the Royal Marsden at Sutton in 2015 when discharged. This was during my 2nd round of chemotherapy treatment. I explained to him, if we could manage my mouth there was a good chance this would keep me from ending up in hospital again. He was receptive to the idea and made sure I had the right medication to help me look after my mouth to prevent me from ending up being admitted. This worked.

April 2016, 6 months post operation, on the home front, I find I still get ulcers from working long hours or eating too late, both actions cause me to have a restless night's sleep. Even a glass of champagne sends me over the edge or an odd coffee cause the same effect. So I try not to do them all at the same time. It is a balancing act. I have to accept if I want to remain in a good state I have to forgo these. With a mouth free of ulcers and pain, it is definitely the right place to be.

The benefits of keeping the mouth moist and clean

The ulcers become less infrequent

Ability to get rid of them quicker

Reduce the discomfort when I have an ulcer

Now I know what triggers my mouth ulcers, how do I go about changing this, do I need to look at what I eat?

Chapter 11:
Changing my eating habits

"In my chosen path of wellbeing my past eating habits did not serve me now"

Thinking back, was I forced to change my eating habits at first when I found out I had cancer? No, it was a combination of situations that changed me, it never really occurred to me nor did I understand that one of the main reasons my immune system was so shot was because of what I was eating, included far too much sugar. Looking back, I realised even my fad diets I had tried hadn't worked and every treat I talked about, was rubbish. I would try to justify why I could have it, because I have been a good person, which was crap. It was all bad. What I am going to share with you here is how I lost 2 stone, 12.70 kilos over 8 months and in the process gained more energy, felt fitter, even during chemotherapy and my hair shone, by changing my diet. It was a big eye opener to learn I was sacrificing my own wellbeing by having lots of desserts which I loved or those Crunchies on Friday. Marshmallows or Jelly Babies were my best buddy whilst sailing and washed down with an abundance of alcohol. The type of cancer I had was fed by sugar. Not good news.

Quote from Coach issue 29, April 27 2016, *"Quick diets don't work, a Danish study has confirmed that there* is no such thing as quick-fix diet. The new research shows that to prevent the pounds piling back on, a diet needs to be followed for a whole year. Crash diets actually increase the levels of hunger hormone, ghrelin, making you want to munch even more than before you started. It takes a whole year of healthy eating to stabilise hunger hormones and make a change this will stick. So if you've only got stamina for three months, don't bother, says science"

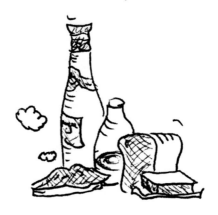

Questions

Can I elaborate on what I used to eat generally in a week?

It is shocking to think I was on a hiding to nothing, knowing what I know of what I did to my poor body, with fad diets on top of what I've mentioned above, and those 'none fat diets'.

OK there were periods when I was in training or my button popped on my trousers which would send me off on a diet. This diet lasted until the trouser button wasn't under pressure allowing me to re-unite my button to my trousers with a few stitches.

Not forgetting I acquired this sweet tooth very early on with my pocket money always going on sweets, this was to the value of sixpence (five new pennies) daily. My taste buds were finely tuned athletes on sweets, my teeth were wrecked, my constant craving for chocolate bars and sugary sweets. Sometimes I would have one of each or devour a whole packet of Jelly Babies. Later when I couldn't eat dairy products I'll opt for alternative, failing to realise they contained high amounts of refined sugars. When I ate sweeties of course I would hide the evidence in the bin so Peter never saw what I was eating. Horrendous thought. All of these contain copious amounts of refined sugar, known to be bad for you if you eat too much, and I did. I was ignorant to how bad what I was eating was for me. All I recognised was what I ate made me fat.

I wouldn't say I was the best cook I, this is where Peter would agree, I had some hits and many misses when it came to cooking. Our diet was normally simple home-made cooking almost every meal was rounded off with a pudding of course. I loved apple crumble, trifles and not forgetting my late mother's Bakewall tart a real treat, (I do have her recipe if you are interested). After dinner, OK almost finished, it would be rounded off with a bit of chocolate before heading to bed. How I slept, God only knows, lots of sex maybe!

I was neither shy of takeaways, or frequenting the local curry house in Ashtead regularly. This is one of my favourite places possibly because Peter proposed to me after dinner at the Mogal. I still smile at the thought of it. What I failed to consider was that it was far too late to digest the meal of that size.

Yes there were fad diets too, no fats, but what I failed to realise was that my diet consisted of too much sugar. Little did I know what I know now, scary thought!

Three times (between the ages of 24 to 45) suffering with suspected appendicitis, in appalling stomach pain, so serious I was admitted into hospital. Each time I remained in for a week, which was followed by an enforced strict diet plan for the next couple of weeks. Everything would then settle down again and I would go back to my good old ways of eating and drinking.

Surprisingly I still have my appendicitis, neither they nor I never got to the root of the problem. It is only now on reflection my body was crying out for a break from gluten or dairy and possibly less sugar and fat. This came to light much later on in 2011 when I was really ill.

There was a sufficient shift in what I ate after returning from Malta in 2011. I was laid up for 10 days very poorly. That was the last time I really could stomach eating dairy or having it in my diet without harsh consequences to my tummy and wellbeing.

I reacted really badly to anything that that had traces of dairy in so I steered far away from it. However, others failed to appreciate how ill I got and felt it was OK to serve me just a little bit in the food. As time went on the side effects got worse, I would feel dreadful, sweating brow, stomach pains, upset tummy for hours, the shoulder pain and no energy. I was in a frightful state, drained exhausted and unable to function for days on end.

As things were starting to get better it all went tits up during my trip to India in 2012. That finished me off, (no dairy ever again). On the last day I ate sushi, come on who eats sushi in India? Raw food, silly me. Well actually that is not entirely true, it was the whole group. I believe I made the homeward bound journey by my quick sense seeking medication at the hotel reception, to my amasement they had a stash of potions in their medicine cabinet. Scary thought, they expected you to get ill.

You wouldn't think it could get worse but it did. After my 2013 chemotherapy treatment my stomach was in absolute turmoil. This was the final straw; my body became even more sensitive and reacted much quicker to any amount of lactose and gluten. I couldn't even cope with a traces of lactose in medication, and now gluten was a no, no. Over the past couple of months since beginning of 2016 I have been able to eat some gluten but find it best not to, as it makes me a bit too regular.

What foods did I eat when I wasn't eating lactose and gluten at first?

Once I removed lactose and gluten from my diet, it took a further 3 years after 2011 to take any further action to as what I ate. OK, I was pretty much eating the same as before whilst excluding foods that contained lactose or gluten. It was crazy, most things I ate either had too much salt or too much refined sugar. It is unreal I didn't look deeper into what I ate at the time.

It is terrible to think, that what my typical diet included daily was a lot of rubbish in 2011. I ate food from the free from range, OK it had no gluten or lactose, but I did not notice there were high quantities of sugar included in these products. Coupled with all this my beverage alcohol consumption was far too high.

On top of everything else I ate and drank, it isn't surprising adding this all up I came crashing down with a big bump.

What where the effects when I ate the wrong thing?

I was constantly tired no energy, ill, restless unable to concentrate, my mind was racing and I was moody, I had many sleepless nights.

WAY FORWARD

My concentration and wellbeing would improve

Look at what I was eating

Introduce fresh alternatives

My weight yo-yoing would become a distant memory

What made me rethink my diet and why?

Eventually I realised in late 2014 all of this was eating away at my immune system, my skin, eyes, hair looked awful, tired and lifeless just because of what I had been eating.

At the start of 2014 I planned to look at creating a better life-style-diet, but it took me until the autumn to do something about it. It was the first time I realised it was my choice to make this change to help manage my mouth and wellbeing through eating the right food. It was not a diet I needed, it was a major overhaul.

Time for a life style check, some dramatic measures were required. I heard myself saying "No Sugar".

Little did I know it would coincide with the news that I had secondary cancer, and receiving sound advice in November from another cancer survivor, Jane. Her experience is a prime example to me. She is now 7 plus years on, well and living a balanced life not only being a wonderful mother but also a successful businesswoman who has created an organic range of skin care products that contain no toxins. She was definitely a person worth listening to.

Since October 2014 I now read every packet of the contents before I buy or eat it. It is far easier to make the meal from scratch. I think Peter noticed my cooking skills got better for a time, when I followed recipes and used my Pure spread and coconut milk instead.

We spoke a few times on the phone and she gave me vast amounts of information, so I made a list of food she recommended me to eat (in the appendix at the back of the book later), and products to use. Still with limited knowledge I wanted to hear more; then amazingly I was introduced to Andrew Hunter, a gift from heaven via Jessica McGregor-Johnson. Andrew had been monitoring his diet for years being a diabetic, and found a way to control his sugars consequently he was free from the symptoms of diabetes. In monitoring his food, he created a diet plan. I was fortunate to be given this diet plan and adopted his guidance via reading what was right and good for my body and mind. I follow his recommendations still to this day.

He said I needed to cut out all refined or residual sugars. It was OK to eat natural sugars; he explained how good sugars came from fresh fruits. It is my goal to keep my refined sugars down to 5% a day and none if possible. The refined sugars are the bad ones for me. Andrew's help was invaluable. Thank you.

Documented from his other guide in "Nancy food update, written by Andrew Hunter in 2014"

"Over the week *- your food should consist of the following and* **in the following proportions**

2%   Meat, lamb – lean (no pork)

3%   Poultry – turkey, then chicken,

5%   Fish

10% Whole grains, almonds, walnuts, flax seeds, sprouts and other sprouting seeds

40% Vegetables ideally raw (with a dip) or steamed – not boiled, fried, etc

40% Fruits,Beans (not baked in sauce) lentils, peas, broad beans, barlotti etc (canned or frozen is fine)"

Basic No Nos and why

Alcohol - likely to contain sugar, yeast, wheat, starch, potatoes

YES red wine seems to get the OK but only a medium glass a day.

Coffee - Small amounts of caffeine in tea or coffee is good for the body and the immune system can deal with this. When you drink more than 2 cups of coffee a day, you expose yourself to large amounts of fungus. Caffeine **acidifies** the blood and tissues which promotes the production of, fungus and mould.

Salt – processed! processed white store bought salt changes the negative charge on the blood cells causing them to stack or combine into symplasts which can lead to oxygen deprivation, congestion, poor circulation, stroke, and/or heart attack.!

YES Use natural sea salt that has had iodine added. Sea salt does wonders for the body and is needed by the body. NB it has to be Celtic sea salt or Himalayan salt.

Sugar (except natural sugar as in fruits and vegetables) - Sugar including honey, maple syrup, corn syrup, high fructose corn syrup, sucrose, rice syrup, barley malt etc. promote the growth of yeast, fungus, and mould and suppress the immune system response up to five hours.

"This guide draws on a philosophy which many complementary therapists believe in:-

Live in harmony with the mind, body, spirit, and emotions and with the natural world in order to achieve a high-level of health and well-being. The approach is threefold.

1. *nourishment through nutrition, looking at the quality and quantity of foodstuffs taken and enhancing the enjoyment of healthy eating, fine-tuned for the individual.*

2. *physical care, eg exercise, breathing, skin care, hydrotherapy and gentle manipulation – gentle massage etc*

3. *psychology or as I like to call it "metaphysics" ie meta – beyond and physics – the physical – un-*

derstanding ourselves and recognising the links between what we think, believe and say, how that affects our emotional states and behaviour patterns and contributes to specific diseases. There is now too much research to ignore."

All of this advice was confirmed when I was at the hospital in January 2015. I was having one of many tests, a PET test where they injected sugar serum into my blood stream. Peter asked why they were doing the test and why the injection? They said "if it was cancer it would feed off the sugar, by reacting to it." When they did the scan it gave them the information they needed to know, it was cancer.

What happened next and the side effects from this strict diet?

The next two months were tough and hard. From October to December 2014, I ate pretty much the same weekly menu plan with guidance from Andrew's document. My weight fell off, I felt and looked good, my hair and eyes started to shine, my energy increased way more than I expected, I noticed my mouth was free of ulcers. But I was scared to deviate off the diet. Other benefits I now could concentrate better, giving me clearer focus on the tasks I was doing *(See appendix 212)*.

Wasn't I the lucky one, to be given such sound guidance of what to eat? Most importantly I chose to listen, and take action. There were times when I was offered a glass of wine in 2014/15, and was tempted to have one. But I resisted. But, I was saddened and scared, with normally a tear in my eye, trying to come to terms with this new life style with so much uncertainty, "saying I want to live, please."

During chemotherapy I had to be more selective in what I eat and drank, this helped me immensely, *(See menu plan page 213, 214 and 215)*. Remembering looking back at the time it was only tough initially because for the past 40 plus years I ate so much rubbish. I did not realise it at the time until months later. The new recipes were easier to make and more enjoyable, and things I thought I would miss, I didn't. Only occasionally I miss Mother's Bakewall Tart. Hey ho. It took me time to gain confidence to explore at other things I could eat. For me I found the health shop a good place to start, I still have a lot to learn to eating the right balance diet over the course of a week.

Great to receive sound advice what to eat

Having more energy during treatment

My eyes and hair shine

I feel more focused and calm

With all this sound advice, what helped me next in my discovery to guide me and help me feel closer to achieving my promise to myself?

Chapter 12:
Pain control, living and managing it

"Can I say pain can magically go away? No. But I have learnt to focus differently so pain didn't control my life."

What I can share is how I changed the energy in my body by removing tension. This in turn reduced and in some instances removed the source of pain totally. My objective is to explain how I was taught to work through pain, helping me to reduce the use of painkillers, whilst keeping sight that the healing process worked faster when I was not in pain. Also, learning to combine the alternative approach alongside the medication pre-scribed by the doctors and consultants; was now the best approach for me during my recovery from surgery and the treatments.

Questions
What was the level of pain was I dealing with?

For me this is the toughest one. I thought right up to having surgery and chemotherapy treatment I had a fairly high threshold of pain, no not at all. What I discovered I could cope with in the past was so different. Here is a prime example of how tough I thought I was, able to sail in the World and national championships for two weeks competing with two broken fingers.

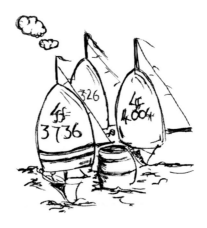

Whilst going though treatment I was struck down in 2013 with a frozen shoulder. The hospital first attempt failed at the Epsom General to free up my frozen shoulder. Without any local anaesthetic, four members held me down then injected a steroid directly in the shoulder, for sure. Boy, did I yell. I can still remember the tears and pain. It was a barbaric procedure, and I told them so. I didn't want another frozen shoulder. After my first operation the pain from that shoulder was horrendous. It took over 6 months to ease up, every moment of the day was exhausting.

Then bang, in 2015 I had the lung operation, this is known as left VATS and segmentectomy surgery. Immediately after this operation I was on a morphine pump, expressing pain relief every 5 minutes. The pain was relentless, I had crossed my threshold of pain, none of the past techniques worked, the pain was unbearable at the time and wore me down. My whole body remained in a state of shock. Any movement was agonising. I sat there frozen to one place in bed and at home scared to move. My thoracic surgeon was great, prescribing me oxycodeine liquid and tablets both of which were a morphine based drug, topped up with lidocaine patches and paracetamol. Yes I was dosed up to the eyeballs. I had some comfort as long as I didn't move. Great, but not great.

Faced with wanting to wean myself off this oxycodone drug as soon as possible, I did it in two stages. First stopping it during the day on week three, I continued with it at night for another 4 weeks. During the first couple of months after the operation sleep never really came into my vocabulary, I had cat naps, through sheer exhaustion. By week three I was getting about 2 or 3 hours sleep a night. Pain was still controlling my life, which was indeed wearing me down body and mind, not a great place to be.

Therefore following my lung operation in 2015, I watched out for any tell tale signs warning me to take it easy. I took great care to look after my shoulders and lung post surgery. I was constantly keeping my shoulder as warm as possible, focused on helping it remain loose and without tension. The moment I noticed those tell tale signs, I changed what I did. It was a bit of a balancing act over two months to keep my shoulder and the side of my body moving without too much pain.

Did the pain stop me from doing things?

Yes, lots of things. I had to accept I couldn't do what I wanted to do. Rather than trying to prove I could, I stopped myself and allowed the pain to subside first. I was very careful and sensible to ask for help; these are a few examples of when I asked for help.

For a couple of weeks my carer helped me get in and out of the bath when I had a shower

Peter placed my sun chair out so I had somewhere to sit during the summer

Peter or the carer made bed

On those times I tried to put my coat on, on my own, I got stuck in some funny and awkward halfway place with my arm stuck up in the air, I definitely need help.

Putting the bin out was a no, no

For quite a few months Henry the Hoover became Peter's best friend

Can I leave you to empty the car?

Making me a drink

Notice the shift, how much better I was getting and what I now needed to ask for help almost a year on

Can you help me pull the boat?

Can you pull in the mainsheet?

If I had a heavy item to move I would look at different ways of moving it, dragging or rolling, rather than lifting it

To open bottles or lid tops or packets, I still find it awkward opening them

Zips and small fittings on the boat, I find it best to get someone else to assist me

I prefer spending my time skiing down a hill rather than having to pole on the flat

I put on an extra thickness of socks so my feet felt more comfortable when I walked

I still have a special duvet underneath my sheet on my bed to help me sleep

To stop them aching I had a special pillow that protects my shoulder so I can rest better at night

I prefer sitting with my legs uncrossed, this is a more comfortable position

The list could go on, I am by no means lazy but have learnt to adapt and stop, as I know when something is too much and I will suffer from doing it later. It is all about getting back to perfect health with little or no pain in the best way.

Who gave me the insights into managing my pain?

Way before this all happened, back in the early 2000's I came across Anna Baldwin, a Transpersonal Psycho-therapist. At the time with an alternative approach to medicine, she helped me through my menopause. She specialised in the Chinese approach, she taught me how to move energy around the body to take away the pain. She reminded me at the time this may take away the pain, but it would not take away the root cause.

During competitive sailing on the race course at the nationals and Worlds, is an example of how I took away the pain in my broken fingers. Just before I went sailing I would sit in a quiet place, were I used her technique called tapping. I would go around my meridian points *(check out the internet to find out more about your own meridian points)*.

Another example of a situation when I used this technique when I couldn't put any pressure on one leg as I had damaged the ligament behind my right knee on the first day of a ten day cycle from Inverness to Petersfield 2010. I was amazed how I could do strenuous exercise after practicing this technique in the morning, so I could remain on my bike day after day, even though at night I couldn't walk on it.

Peter was due to join me for dinner that evening on the 9th day of this stage, and if he knew how much pain I was in when I stopped cycling he wouldn't have let me carry on. I used her technique again, on my last night before stopping to meet Peter. I had cycled over 80 miles that day. So I thought, OK I have used the technique during the day, maybe I could extend it to incorporate the evening as well. True to form, that night I could walk without a limp or any pain. It was incredible what you can achieve if you put your mind to it. The great thing was he was none the wiser that I had damaged my ligament. It was only a day later he was aware when he saw how painful it was for me to walk on it. He made me rest for two weeks before I was allowed back on my bike.

It took until another 5 years later in 2015 at The Royal Marsden on the private wing, for a nurse who specialised in pain control to explain to me the best way to manage my pain at a higher level. Funny, it wasn't rocket science. She made me see that late at night my pain would be at its worst. This was because the brain was channelling all thoughts and energy towards the pain, a survival instinct of the body to help repair it, but actually all it was doing was in-tensifying the tension creating more pain, which was actually slowing down the repairing process of the body. Highlighting the fact that the longer I stayed still, the pain would intensify, contrary to previous medical advice of years gone by.

With that in mind I had to change my thought process, I watched TV, or read a book, get up and walk around anything that would distract my mind. That was the first step in the right direction to help me control my pain. OK it didn't take away the pain totally but it had the good result of helping me cut down on my drugs after the D flap breast surgery quicker than after the VATS Lung surgery. OK let's not forget the severity of the pain. Both times I was on a morphine pump for the first 3 days. This was a big breakthrough for me. Now, almost a year on, when I am in pain, I get up and move around first. It is great, I haven't taken a painkiller for months.

Other techniques for removing the pain came from seeing Tony in early April 2015. I still found some of the methods weird, but lo and behold, every time I asked him to help take away the pain, he was as good as his word and did it. On one occasion it was like watching one of those witch doctors wiggling a small smouldering stick smoking over my shoulder, I felt a harsh intense pain then the pain suddenly vanished. He didn't touch me, it was a bit like magic. He hasn't done that since, but he been great at topping up my energy levels at each of the remainder of the sessions.

WAY FORWARD

Having a different approach to doing things

Asking for help

Recognising my limitations and having fun in the process

Distracting the mind from pain

In the early stages in 2012 of my treatment in 2012 I lived in fear. There were a few things that triggered me to worry.

Heart racing

It was when my heart was racing I had silly thoughts that my heart wasn't right, I realise now it was heightened by the chemotherapy injection and remained like that for a few days. I was worried as I was aware of the side effects caused by the treatment which could weaken the heart.

Head and body aching

When I was hospitalised with low neutrophils my body ached. I was exhausted and scared I could end up with an infection which my body was not equipped to cope with.

Stories I heard of pulling stitches

One of my friends told me her story of when she went sailing and ended up having to retie some of her stitches whilst out sailing in the Solent. This put me off a bit. The idea of my wound opening up was scary to imagine. Yes, horrible thought, because I was sensitive to glues and dressing they omitted placing any dressing on my my wounds other then one very small plaster.

Not knowing what to expect post op

I recall, after the surgery on the right breast on a wide local excision and axillary node clearance to remove DCIS with isolated tumour cells plus 20 lymph nodes in February of 2013, the physiotherapist said I should expect discomfort initially when I started do stretching. This really scared me with thoughts of my friend in mind. I was a National Health patient at the time and looked after absolutely perfectly. An array of physiotherapy stretching exercises were given to me in the form of a booklet, with time lines of when I could do x y and z, so I followed the timelines and exercise to the letter, once I was given a little nudge by the nurse.

Pain of frozen shoulder

The one thing that held me back was the frozen shoulder. No amount of exercise helped, it took time and special hands. I am still wary of my shoulder now and listen to it. When it starts to ache I stop there and then what I am doing, or change the exercise to be kinder to myself.

Aching muscles

I had a persistent nagging leg pain for far too long, no amount of painkillers would take away the aching muscles and sore bones. It wasn't until October 2014 that I was introduced to Jane Dovey Chartered Physiotherapist, Grad Dip Phy MCSP who had gone down the route of homeopathic remedies, via Kirsty Apthorp. Up to then I would have been more cautious and scared I could break something if I did too much when I had those aches.

Not knowing my limits

Let me fast forward to May 2016 and testing my limits. Taking all the above into account it is still a balancing act not to overdo it. I thought I knew my limits. The absence of aching muscles and bones is a great feeling. However, I still go off for a few days to rest up when I get a ulcer, scared of the consequences if I do not pay attention to these reminders.

Able to manage my pain with ease

Using alternative approach

Trusting in different methods

Recognising my limitations has put me in a good place

Pain did control my life but once I gained an understanding it didn't have to stop me from doing things, what would I have to accept next in my life should I choose to change?

Chapter 13:
Sleeping pattern change during treatment

"Nothing prepared my mind physically or mentally for the restless nights and the hours awake. Somehow the body is amazing and how it adapts so quickly to cope"

I had no idea the simple thing I took for granted of 8 hours sleep every night was going to suddenly become a faded distant memory 2012. My body did not do what it would normally do, to slip into a nice deep sleep at night anymore. This was possibly the most challenging time, at night when I was alone, tired and unable to control the body. Too much was happening to allow me to be comfortable when I slept, the aching legs, the wriggling feeling, the hot flushes, the heart pounding, the nausea, my foul taste buds, my sore tongue, high temperatures, the dryness, the pain from the surgery and when I was crying out for sleep my scar tissue continued to keep me awake since 2013. Not to mention the mental and physical strain placed on me having to accept this was something I have to learn to adapt to; rest when I can and count my blessings. To date my nights are broken but I have learnt to live with it. Let me tell you how I coped with the loss of a good night's sleep to carry on a normal life.

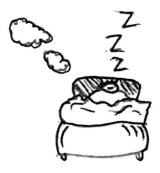

Questions

How did I manage when I had no sleep at night?

I didn't cope at all well at the beginning. Thrashing around in the bed and becoming tense didn't help the cause at all. For the first few weeks in 2012, I believed this was a temporary thing and I could put up with it, like getting better, over a period of 6 weeks, I thought it would subside then go away.

So after a few weeks I recognised if I lay still as much as I could and rested then that must surely be doing me some good in some form or other. It seemed to work for a while. I did lots of cap naps at first. Most of them strangely were during the day. Few were by night.

I couldn't at first get myself to sleep when I was in so much pain. However, I rested in bed reading, but when my eyes were too tired looking at the words, I watched a fun video on my laptop.

What techniques have I put in place to help me have a better night's sleep?

What normally helped me was a warm glass of coconut milk with banana mixed together. This normally gained me two more hours sleep.

When my body had the chemotherapy drug racing around it first in 2012, then 2015, to calm it down I drank more water. This helped, reducing that sensation of bubble bees buzzing around my body, but caused me to visit the loo more, the better of two evils.

The yoganedra technique sometimes worked for about an hour. Between midnight and three am were the worst times, back to a glass of milk.

As the weeks became months, I took to meditating when I went to bed. I still do this technique now, especially when I feel tired. This normally sends me to sleep for a good couple of hours.

I find having an active day helps, again a bit of balancing act. A good walk out helps me sleep well.

I found not having such a heavy meal in the evening helped me, opting for a nice hearty lunch instead.

I seldom have real coffee, and when I do I generally have it no later than mid morning. That seems to work.

Refined sugars are an absolute no, no for me, I monitor this daily on everything I eat to keep it to about 5 grams max, or none at all if possible. It is surprising how many products' ingredients include those refine sugars. Opting to feel calm this has been a real win to exclude sugar from my diet this helps me sleeps.

Not looking at the computer or mobile phone during the couple of hours before bed.

Having a nice cup of lavender tea before bed helps me settle down.

I find turning down the lights works. Softer light just before getting ready for bed helps me settle quicker.

Refraining from having a bath to late in the day, as the hot water stimulates the nerve and would keep me awake.

WAY FORWARD

Be kinder on my body

Eat lighter meals

Create a calmer environment prior to going to bed

Settle down in bed even if I couldn't sleep

Look at alternative approaches

What benefits did I get from meditation in preparation for sleep and coping with what has happened over the past four years?

In a few words there were lots.

Calmer

Centred

Balanced

Healthier

It is great I feel this way it has created a perfect way forward for me in my journey of choices.

Understand the benefits of resting

Sleep helped my recovery

Enjoy the comfort of resting when not sleeping

Good hearty walk helps during the day, aids my sleep

That leads me on nicely to what is the next step of making a promise to myself, I chose to look at exercise.

Chapter 14:
The benefits of outside exercise

"For me nature grows in many different forms and shapes, I feel the natural fresh air allows me to connect with new energy, when I exercise outside"

I have found that taking in fresh oxygen pulls in goodness, this I feel has aided my healing process quicker and given me new energy to enjoy activities each day. My objective is to share how being outside exercising daily, over the last couple of years, by taking long walks has brought me to a place where I can comfortably go for a run or go skiing, cycling and sailing, which are three of my passions.

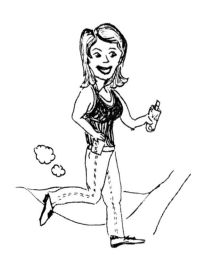

Questions

How fit would I describe myself?

I would say I am generally fitter than most people. That is still not a sensible or correct answer, hmm. Difficult to quantify fit. I have always been active, not fit. For a start, look at what I was eating in the past. Now, OK what I eat has really changed. You could say I am now getting fit for the first time, yes learning to adapt in a slow, balanced way to getting fit. Why? Because I need to learn first to listen to my body, in reducing my tiredness and building up my stamina, then I will get fit.

Fitness for me isn't only physical. It is balance of both physical and mental awareness dealing with the challenges life has thrown at me. During chemotherapy treatment, especially the first round in 2012, my mind became fuzzy, a light-headed feeling all the time, horrible and scary. It took immense effort to process information or to find answers which were normally readily available, which now were somewhere lost in my head. There were times I wasn't even able to audibly answer a question, or hear what someone was saying. More than exhausting, it was a scary feeling. I lost not only my physical fitness but also my mental fitness at the same time.

Why and what were the reasons for doing it?

So faced with the inability physically and mentally to operate, why did I want to get outside during my first round of chemotherapy in 2012, but seldom did? When I did, it lifted my spirit, I did find walking enjoyable.

Having spent so much time indoors in 2012-13, during the summer months of 2014 it was my choice to spend more time outside. The most effective way was taking longer walks at the weekends. I looked at extending my distances to include walking a marathon over a day with dear friend Gillian. OK I had sore feet blisters and my legs hurt, but I came off quiet well surprisingly, (possibly a bit extreme). It is great now to look back on how far I achieved that summer.

I did recognise I lost the ability to concentrate after my second operation in January 2015. It could have been amplified because of the pain in the side by my lung then I had to endure 6 weeks' chemotherapy. This rather finished me off, I felt totally wasted. I pushed myself to remain as much as possible in a normal daily routine for mental and physical stimulation, like washing up, reading a newspaper, doing a crossword, doing a few jigsaw puzzles, only watching TV after 12:30 when I took lunch, this routine really helped. I generally took a stroll after lunch.

Moving on to the autumn of 2015 with the noticeable changes in my diet I felt stronger, with more energy. On a weekend in February 2016 I chose to walk further, still recognising I had dips in my energy levels. At the half way point after 3 plus miles, the watering hole was a perfect place to re-energise myself, a welcome stop. Preceding this walk I frequently returned spent of energy, retiring to the sofa for the remainder of the day. Now 7 months on walking has becoming pleasurable again, rather than just an exercise.

Then came the third operation looming in June 2015. I knew my fitness level was spent already. After the last operation, I understood and worked out not to push beyond my limitations, therefore chose to do things with a different approach, slowly, slowly catchee monkey, starting my exercise little by little. By the end of the summer months I saw some improvement in my body and mind. Things I had lost in my head started filtering back. I found I was mentally fitter than I thought possible, this was a great place to be.

It was good to see that by putting a fitness programme in place it is starting to pay off. My energy levels are more stable than in the early days when my energy would without warning disappear. It is great I am now hankering to get back on my bike. This is somewhere in my mind I haven't been for a long time.

My sofa days are becoming less frequent because I have understood the importance of listening to my body constantly. I know I still have a long way to go before I am at the fitness level that I would like to be at, but I am in a very good place right now today in May 2016.

BENEFITS

Putting a programme in place helped me

I was aware of my body constrains during treatment and recovery

Measure and control energy levels better

Keep myself mentally and physically stimulated

Was it easy to go and do exercise?

Let me share the issues I faced over the couple of years coping with all this. After the first operation in 2013 I lacked confidence, I therefore found it rather difficult to go outside the door. It took a lot of mental attitude was required. Strange really, once I got outside, past the front door, it was always an enjoyable experience taking a walk. At the beginning I would push myself to walk a mile 3 times a week. During the period of the first couple of weeks post operation, my shoulder hurt more than the breast, my armpit was tight but not too un-comfortable. They told me the stiffening of the shoulder was caused by two things, the amount of time my arm had been raised above my head during the operation, plus the shock of actually having the operation itself and the drugs.

Then I had an awful setback, a frozen shoulder in April 2013. I could do nothing, because I couldn't physically move it. The pain drained me mentally. I tried in vain to get it to move including a daily ritual of physiotherapist stretching. All went to pot just because I almost fell down the stairs grabbing out to catch the handrail and in the process jarred my shoulder. The pain was excruciating. No amount of physiotherapy or alternative approaches worked, it remained frozen and painful for months. Every day I religiously heated it, over the coming months I lived on tramadol constantly in pain. Nothing would budge it, I couldn't move without pain. One of the most awful period of my life not finding anything easy.

Still with limited exercise the next four months were painfully slow, my shoulder complaining all the time. I disciplined myself to stick to the walking. Bearing in mind any sudden movement during the walk, like stepping awkwardly off a curb, would send shooting pains around my body, telling me in no uncertain terms not to move. Boy there were many teary moments.

The exercise got back on track and become easier once again after undergoing a 2nd procedure by Dr George at Epsom General to relieve the frozen shoulder, a gift from heaven. He carried it out under the guidance of a CT scan to inject a steroid in my shoulder, first administering me with an anaesthetic, to numb the area. With this in mind Carina Petter, Osteopath, Pediatric Osteopath, Cranial Osteopath D.O; D.P.O; MSCC, choose the techniques that felt most appropriate for me at the time, this of which she selected from had a wide variety of techniques available in the 'tool kit' in this case she choose using Cranial technique Little by little the movement came back gradually. Softly, softly I stretched and increased my exercise to loosen it up further. With lots of warm showers, hot water bottles, special pillows and a scarf wrapped around my arm and shoulder keeping it snug and cosy all the time, it took 4 months to recover, including a daily routine of yoga. Stretching it helps and still when it gets cold I have to remember to wrap it up or it starts to give me warning signals. During these 4 months no exercise was easy. I had that feeling of lack of energy, like I was walking in mud.

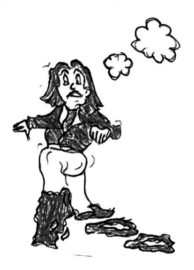

The shoulder started feeling better in late 2013 when I took up swimming at the local swimming baths the Mountbatten centre. The only reason was because the air and water temperatures were warmer indoor pool (for those who don't know me I prefer swimming in the sea than a pool). I did swim once or twice in the sea, well floated really, my front crawl stroke was wonky to say the least, but it did not deter me from trying. With limited movement I knew it was doing me good keeping it moving. The difficulty for me was I was still scared I might hurt it if I tried to move it too much. I didn't know my limitations or how much my shoulder wanted to move and how it would react to too much coldness from swimming in the sea. I definitely didn't want a recurrence of a frozen shoulder again. All these limitations were new ground for me, a big balancing act over those months.

A sense of light relief came in the September, the welcome news I was fit enough to travel. La Manga here I come. This was a big turning point to exercise in the luxury of Spanish sun. The pool became my best friend over that week spending most of my time splashing around and working on getting full movement back in my shoulder, without even really realising.

Then the uncertainty, yes lacking confidence to get back on my bike. It was way into the late summer of 2014, a 12 month gap in total. With my shoulder working again, I started out gradually first heading off to the local shops, then venturing further afield to Mengham the Island's main shopping centre about 20 minutes each way. It should have been frustrating but I strangely accepted that in my past were faded memories to savour and in my future goals to work towards. At this moment in time I had to settle for the short rides, as I knew my limitations, still being drained of energy. To help make trips out on my bike more pleasurable, I took to cycling the seafront route, taking in sights of the boats bobbing up and down in Hayling Bay, on the east side of the Solent entrance.

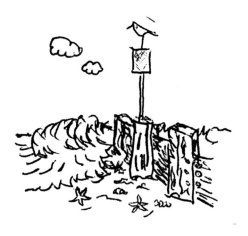

It was hard contemplating our scheduled ski trip in early January 2014. This was a tough thought, would I be able to ski after all I had been through? Bearing in mind I wasn't fit, my legs still ached and I got tired quickly. Hmm. Here is an account of what happened on the first day out skiing. When I put pressure on my inside ski edge my bones and muscles ached they felt like they were going to explode and break. Boy they were sore. I remember the first couple of runs, I felt sad, thinking is every day I ski now is it going to be the same, will I ever be able to ski without pain and enjoy it as much as

I did before? Oh what an awful thought, if I can't. At the time Peter and his two boys were great, truly supportive. They were unaware how I was thinking, but possibly they could see it in my facial expressions or quietness.

This was a hard reality check. I was beating myself up and that was silly. What I failed to remember or consider was that had I just had chemotherapy treatment, topped off with an operation and radiotherapy and a frozen shoulder. All this had wiped me out totally, mentally and physically. And there was I expecting my heart and muscles to take this level of pressure without complaining, was I mad? I had not done any real exercise for over a year other than walking and popping out to the local shops on my bike, get real. Skiing is possibly one of the most physical exercises I could do, together with the cold climate and altitude. I recognised I should not beat myself up. I continued skiing the morning disheartened, calling it a day at 2pm after lunch.

A different mental approach was needed setting out on day 2. Having to walk down to the slope helped me warm up my body. I was determined to get this cracked, first a series of stretching exercises helped. I think the boys understood how tiring it was for me from the day before's performance. Richard offered to carry my skis. I was touched when he said, "well you used to always carry our skis when we were little boys, it's our turn to help you." It made me cry with pride, it still bring tears to my eyes writing it. It was a very special moment, I felt blessed. Now on the slope I thought it best to do turns that used the minimum effort, using a long sweeping turning technique to start with. I had to give it another shot, if I hadn't I'm not sure if I would be skiing now. I was careful to pick only to ski on a well groomed piste, I repeated the same run 3 more times the guys loved blasting down it. What I noticed was my aches were becoming less and less, the aches in my bones felt bearable. I noticed the reduction of pressure I was beginning to feel less scared and more confident each run, I was going to crack this and I wasn't going to break anything. Each run got better. I erred on the side of caution that day and stopped shortly after lunch counting my blessings. A perfect second day, I celebrated in Ku De Ta with Peter, Simon and Richard, my boys.

Day by day skiing for me was getting easier on my body. I got over confident skiing off-piste doing turns in the deep powder. However, not noticing, and misjudging a ridge on re-entering the piste where there was a step up not down. It knocked me off guard and I did this amazing head plant right by Peter's feet ending in a heap, dazed and with a sore thumb. Come the next day I happily enjoyed a sofa day reading a book and cooking the evening dinner and nursing my sore thumb. A reminder of my limitations.

Out skiing a few days on with my thumb strapped up, it was just great to be back in the mountains with Peter and the boys, Simon and Richard. We had an amazing ski holiday. I was well on the way to getting fitter. This ski trip opened up new opportunities mentally and physically. We laughed a lot and life was less scary. The holiday was another milestone on the road to learning my limitations and I thoroughly enjoyed every moment back on my skis.

Now refreshed, confident and happy I could increase my exercise daily. By the spring I was back in the boat, it was surprisingly easy climbing back into it. It felt like I had never been out of it. Subsequently we went on to sail in the Bulwark open meeting at my club and I was delighted to achieved another one of my goals sailing in the Nationals at Parkstone Yacht Club in 2014. Two great weekends. I truly appreciated being at the start line but I knew my limitations, we were not competitive if it blew above a force 2, we had a few good results and enjoyed the hospitality of the committee boat watching the fleet when tired.

After going from 80 kilos to 70 kilos to help place the weight right in the boat we swapped places in the October 2014. We agreed I was better helming the boat leaving Peter to do the physical stuff as the crew. This worked for a while. However I know Peter was frustrated crewing for me.

In the November all sports almost stopped, when I was diagnosed with a recurrence of cancer in my right breast. I awaited news of when I was to have a lung operation. I was hesitant to do too much exercise in fear of what the side effects would be if I did too much physical sport, so I decided to curtail my sailing and opt only for walking, with an occasional sail on light air days.

This was hardest mentally for me, this waiting game for tests and getting time to see the consultants was painful. In need of a distraction I was delighted to be given the green light to head off for a last minute ski holiday to Wengen for Christmas. I was rather unsure at first, thinking that the activity of skiing, coupled with altitude, could hurt my lung or cause the cancer to grow more. I had no idea what would happen, so I skied with caution at first, soon distracted when we joined up with the Ski guide from the Ski Club of Great Britain plus a couple of members who had invited us from the Downhill Only Club in Wengen. I suddenly had lots of energy, far more than expected. It was a wonderful feeling being back skiing. The love of the mountains, my passion to be back on skis gave me moments when I forgot there was anything wrong Yes, I was tired but this was because of the uncertainty of the coming months and what lay ahead. I did find it hard to relax when I wasn't skiing, and felt like I was wasting time rather than enjoying every moment. The holiday lined me up perfectly for the next few months.

I was so lucky that I had the best surgeon to remove the singular lump from my left lower lung, known as a VATS procedure, in January 2015. After my previous breast operation two years before, I had expected to be sore for the first few days post operation but this was different, I could not describe the pain, all I could say it was relentless, it hurt me to move let alone exercise for many weeks.

It was all I could do to get myself in and out the shower with the aid of a carer. To drag myself out the front door seem impossible, with the help of the carer my first walk consisted of a stroll around the close car park all of 100 metres but the first step in the right direction. The pain prevented me from wanting to move and I felt scared I might hurt or damage myself even more if I tried to push it.

January 2015 That first few weeks post op, were emotionally hard. I was feeling tentative and unsure with every movement, bearing in mind I was on two types of *morphine drugs*. I was on foreign ground experiencing such discomfort, it hurt, it was gruelling, this was horrible and scary and I hated those weeks. Nothing was enjoyable; there were no rewards other than more pain. But slowly each day I set new targets to reach, and failed daily over the coming month. On day 4 I made one of my markers. I remember walking all the way across the common with a smile, a good 800 yards, to the doctors surgery, my whole body shaking with exhaustion. I had no idea how I was going to get myself home I dragged my body home to the comfort of the sofa and bed for the remainder of the day. It took 6 weeks of help from the carer and Peter before I could move my body. As the weeks went by I started to appreciate the walks once again.

After the recovery from surgery it was hard to think I still had 4 sessions of chemotherapy to go through. During the previous treatment I had been really ill, but I felt the new diet and the logging of what foods and exercise I could do during the 21 day cycle the time before might stand me in good stead. It did. (See the menus, energy and how I felt on page 214 and 215).

With this plan, prior to heading off to the hospital for my first round of chemotherapy injection in the April 2015. I prepared the fridge with water with cucumber and hint of ginger. I went for a walk that morning, knowing when I got back I would need to rest and have to drink lots of water, (which I still do today). I continued walking daily. I only stopped if absolutely wasted. During treatment I walked 15 days out of the 21 day cycle which really helped me physically and mentally. During the treatment the oncologist and I became close and we talked a lot. I coped better this time around. This was due to the exercise, food, right mouth management, mental support and rest and the attention to detail of my consultants and doctors. Support was second to none, thank you.

Chemotherapy completed I was scheduled to have another operation in the June. A respite was desperately needed. My body had been battered and bruised in the past months, it was time to relax and have fun in the company of Peter and my dear friends Nick and Jayne, I got the go ahead to have a week sunning myself in Spain at La Manga once again. The warmth of the sun was a blessing. This news was a gift from heaven knowing I would be swimming and walking.

Whilst there we took to Nordic walking. This 3 miles seemed like a stroll in the park whilst we walked and talked. The advantage was I was able to spend more time in the pool than out, which was a refreshing way to energise whilst building up my stamina, which helped me physically and mentally for my next round of operations. I must say this time all my activities were easy and enjoyable, the right way to exercise. I had a lot of fun playing pitch and putt, to my amusement I won most of the rounds. The evenings I relaxed in their company playing bridge or sitting down and watching videos, a truly enjoyable week's distraction.

On returning from holiday feeling pretty fit physically and mentally, I was definitely in the right mind set as I could ever be for this D flap operation to my right breast. I also made before the operation a conscious decision that it was time I set some targets to help me keep focused.

Uncertain how I was going to achieve this, I got some great outside assistance from Tony J. Selimi, who got me to focus on how I should map out my time lines to work towards actually achieving these actions. I had a few things I wanted to accomplish and be comfortable in doing them. They included such as: Simple things I took for granted.

Walk in standing upright when I went to see my consultant after the operation on the 9th day

Sitting in a car for up to 4 hours

Walking a good couple of miles whilst retaining some energy for later

Being able to organise Peter's party in October

Be focused to work for an 8 hour day

This was my first stepping stone, was it going to be easy? Hmm.

Each of these actions I wanted to achieve had their own issues and were hard to contemplate and possibly harder had I set them post op, but because I set them beforehand it had helped as I knew from my previous operations my schedule of recovery was about 6 to 7 weeks if all went well.

June 2015 first I set about some simple slow stretching exercises to my body to stand upright whilst taking a very slow walk around the garden. I spent most of the day outside reading, enjoying the warmth of the sun and relaxing in the shade. Popping in and out to get a few bits, I was left to fend for myself possibly sooner than I wished, but in the end it was good for me. Mark my word with the first goal ticked off, walking upright (this wasn't easy, as my sister described me as walking like my mother in her failing years), I was on to the next one.

I took to lengthening my walks daily. Within the coming weeks I was up to walking around the park in Ashtead by week three. I looked at increasing my stretching. It became more comfortable sitting upright longer, (it is still uncomfortable today 10 months on if I remain in the same position for too long). I knew I was progressing much better than after my earlier operation in the year as I had greater movement with less discomfort. Yes it was painful, but bearable. Maybe being shown how to focus on removing this pain by movement contributed to this. I talk about that elsewhere in this book, and about the many nights of sleeplessness, some call it sleep deprivation too.

With my targets clearly set, knowing I needed to do both sitting for a long period of time and walking for a good mile, with my pending journey travelling by ferry and car mid August to join up with Peter in Crozon Morget. The idea was also to see friends and fellow sailors competing at the Flying Fifteen World Championship. The time line was tight but achievable, a comforting thought.

Each day I increased my time spent walking, stretching and sitting rather than lying. This was helped by taking trips out on the train to see the consultant rather than getting a lift in a car or taking a taxi.

With less than 2 weeks before my French trip I was determined to see how I would fare on a day out. The idea was a dress rehearsal, this was my big first outing where I would mingle in large crowds, with lengthy times standing around and walking. I had planned to be with Steve and Alison my in-laws to watch the America's Cup World Series in Portsmouth 2016. We arranged to meet in Havant and catch the train. The idea was to have a lot of fun, indeed on the day it was cut short because the race was blown off but it didn't dampen our spirits. The atmosphere on the train was brilliant, everyone chatting in the carriage regardless if you knew them, we were all so excited. That day I got to see Team BAR crew packing up their craft AC45F in their headquarters located at Spice Island. The whole place was buzzing, I felt blessed to be there, we finished off the day having fish and chips at the Still and West overlooking the sights of the harbour and Portsmouth Historic Dockyard. A magical day had by all.

At the same time I was pleased that the consultant was carefully monitoring my progress, he gave me the OK to drive a week earlier than expected. Great news, this opened up the opportunity to head down to Hayling Island and spend a few days chilling out on the beach before my next adventure across the channel. Mindful that my tummy was still very tender when I touched, I decided to drive with a pillow tucked between the safety belt strap. The idea was to make myself as comfortable as possible. This worked well all the time as a passenger, so no harm for me doing it as a driver I thought. During the few days spent at Hayling I went for a dip in the sea, rather chilly, cannot call it swimming, but enjoyably refreshing. I believe salt water has healing qualities, well that is what I believe.

I was apprehensive a few days before heading off to France, in need of distraction. My friend Sue Parkin came to the rescue, she had flown in and wanted to catch up with old friends and had arranged a special dinner. Both Jan and I went. It was great to be included the food and service was appalling hey ho never mind. (There is an opportunity there for someone to go in and make this restaurant a great place).

Early start on D day, we took 5 hours on the crossing from Portsmouth to Caen, plus a further 5 hours in the car driving down to the most-loveliest of welcomes. We arrived to see Peter's smiley face greeting us at the quay of Crozon Morget. I had an amazing few days amongst friends sitting on the quayside lapping up the sun, smiling and feeling really happy walking the beach with Peter. I reached my second and third targets, yippee. I felt blessed, OK sore and uncomfortable, but putting that aside it was great to be there for a wonderful few days with friends and hubby in France. Than you Fran for taking us to the ferry.

The year held lots of lovely trips, they all aided my recovery. This included an outing with Peter to Sete, a delightful small coastal fishing port in the south of France. Whilst there I felt I regained a lot of energy. This I put down to focusing very much on the actions I did daily and staying away from any distractions. The great thing was we pretty much had a normal holiday. I swam in the sea, though I must say it was a bit nippy (Hayling Island surprisingly is warmer). I didn't hang around in the water for long, preferring to spend the weekend taking in the sights, walking and talking, we walked a good 3 miles each day, very relaxing. Yes I was tired my muscles complained at night keeping me awake. I was still opting for early nights, heading to bed by 9:30 pm. It was a great few days break. I remember Peter saying to me "I feel I have my Susan back." That brought tears of happiness to my eyes.

In mid October 2015 a short break from exercise came when I had the cosmetic operation to "tidy up the dog ends" as my consultant described it. It stopped me for a few weeks until I had my stitches out. However, with discomfort and lack of sleep I continued with my walking. I was surprised how painful it was when my clothes rubbed my stomach and sides, (my nerves continued to be over sensitive and still are 6 months on if I wear something tight around my waist). It prevented me from doing anything strenuous. However, it still didn't stop me from having fun dancing at Peter's party a week after the operation with my two sisters, what a great evening.

I was surprised how much that operation zapped my energy, but putting that all aside I was only bruised and had pretty much had full movement as long as I didn't touch my sides or stomach. The breast was OK, I didn't really notice that discomfort just the strange lack of feeling. All I had to do was be careful not to bang my body or let anyone touch or hug me for a couple of months, I could put up with that. I was back to sleep deprivation, but I got used to that I had learnt to sleep on my back with a padded duvet underneath me. This is the most comfortable way to sleep.

With skiing after Christmas in my sights I recognised I was a long way from being fit for that amount of activity, hmm. Fortunately a day later I bumped into my Pilates teacher on the train. Fiona turned out to be a blessing, a great find. Bit of luxury having a private lesson, yes I know, it was the only way I knew I would get fit in time without damaging myself. I feared with my competitive streak, if I joined a class I would be the one too eager to be doing it right and miss something and hurt myself in the process. But by having an eagle eye watching and checking me I would have to do it right. I hadn't really realised how beneficial the art of Pilates is when you engage the right muscles for the various exercises. Her one to one tuition was perfect. I was pleased to gain so much more stamina from doing Reformer Pilates. Each session my core was getting stronger.

Two weeks before skiing I felt fit enough to go for two runs, I upped-the-anti with swimming too. I noticed that back stroke was hardest for me 11 months on after my lung operation and still caused me some discomfort and restricted movement but I kept working at using my arms. I pushed myself too hard, paying the price a few days later when I got an ulcer in my mouth. I had to slow down again. Achieving the fine balance was difficult for me but I had to recognise and understand my limits.

Guess what? Skiing in late January was awesome. I appreciated that spending the months before slowly building the programme of exercise, had paid off. Lots of powder off-piste, lots of energy, skied most days for about 4 hours, it was fantastic. As you can see, setting goals is worth it, thanks to you Tony, Fiona, and my consultants. It was my choice to take action, bless everyone along the way for giving insight and encouragement. It was made even better having the time with dear friends from Hayling, team Chalet thank you, Anna, Angus, John, Chris and lovely Peter for a great holiday.

Though still not firing on all cylinders I must remember not to beat myself up too much. Cycling has been the only thing I haven't really done much of, OK I have been on the bike a bit. It may have been one of the wettest, windiest winters, roll on summer, I might get to pump up my tyres soon, I did go out one late May 2016 sunny day and thoroughly enjoyed the cycle.

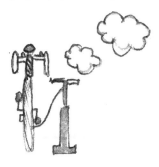

Some reflections and thoughts about exercise

Long before my first operation I happily stretched as a matter of course to remain supple. It was in the past 4 years all new territory, I was finding it hard to contemplate doing exercise during the past couple of years, let alone actually do the stretching in the first place. I remember thinking, I have to have some self discipline here. This is how I started. First thing in the morning in the shower when the room was hot, I set a target to stretch up my arms to see if I could touch the ceiling. Prior to that I would roll my arms up the side of the wall and see how high I could get them up each time, looking to get them higher each time. Then when I had finished in the shower, another simple task of scrapping the wall was required. A bit like karate kid exercise, I worked out that scraping down the water off the tiles would help me stretch my shoulder, arms and torso. A simple task, initially I remember it being hard. The great thing is I would have a shower daily so this was a great way of starting to get my movement back. I could see the progress.

I recall in 2015 they hadn't offered any physiotherapy but I think my consultants recognised I had more than enough self discipline, setting my own physiotherapy programme, to be in charge of getting my movement back. I received very encouraging words to hear coming from the nurses and the consultants "you are far fitter than most of our other patients."

I was conscious I needed to concentrate on the other actions. If I wished to work for more 8 hour stretches, bearing in mind I know I didn't fare well after attending an hours' meeting early on after my operations, I now had to focus on the best way this could be achieved. I had to lengthen my concentration, so in the day I would set simple tasks that included doing a puzzle, seeing if I could do a crossword. Other tasks included reading a book, stimulating my brain was one of the key factors in my recovery. Improving my French and Italian linguistic skills was also on my agenda, and still is, by learning a word of each on most days.

My explanation has been rather lengthy; indeed it is hard both mentally and physically but I am finding it worth it in the long run. All the time in the past I never considered what I did was exercise, just fun stuff, doing pleasurable things filled my life. I always enjoyed swimming in the sea, sailing, cycling, skiing and stretching, why should I consider it hard to do? It is only now when my body aches that I realise that there is a reason getting fit is called exercise. Something I have to get used to.

How did I select my exercises and when I did them?

My selection of exercises came from outside influences. Thelma Cooper, a Physiotherapist subscribed me to VITA, a magazine for breast cancer sufferers and survivors. I found the magazine rather down trodden and seldom picked it up to read it. However, on rare occasions I came across an interesting article backing up the reasoning behind Thelma's recommendations for exercise. That gave me a kick start to walk during chemotherapy treatment. It was my aim to walk daily for about 20 minutes. I benefitted from these lovely walks, ambling up through the private lanes leading on to Ashtead common whilst chatting to the birds and horses on the way. Some of the mornings I dragged myself out, the whys and wherefores I have touched on elsewhere in these pages. The idea was to stop me sitting around and allow me to build up stamina, increase my fitness and reduce the risk of blood clots whilst taking gentle exercise.

I was sent home after my first surgery on my breast and lymph nodes in 2013 with guidelines mapped out in a booklet confirming what series of stretches I needed to do, these were more generic physiotherapist exercises with set time lines of when I should be able to regain the full range of movement of my right arm and shoulder without putting too much load on them during the recovery period.

It was my choice to have some control over what I included. I started to keep a chart to see if there were windows when my energy levels were at their best during the course of 8 cycles of chemotherapy treatment, to notice the highs and lows. The chart gave me some control of different aspects of my life, when it was OK to have a day out, knowing my body was in a good shape to do that.

The Royal Marsden offered a great rehabilitation centre which provided 6 free sessions to various classes for physical and mental benefit, so I decided to take up their offer. I enrolled to pamper myself with a series of massages, as well as taking a few private relaxation sessions. Never did the massages or the relaxation sessions work for me, the massage maybe because it caused me to dip too low in energy afterwards which made me feel dreadfully ill. However, the relaxation sessions were more like a counselling session; her voice didn't work for me. I suppose I realise now thinking back how thankful I am for this opportunity to have had these sessions. At the time I was too locked up in my own scared thoughts so I stopped short of completing the course of sessions, maybe because what I really needed was a session to share my thoughts.

Then came the yoga classes at The Royal Marsden in Sutton. I had this idea that after the class it would be a bit of a social and we would all go off and have coffee and share our thoughts. However the others, all with their own problems possibly, kept themselves to themselves. I wasn't getting any social benefit from attending so I felt after attending two sessions I would be better off doing this yoga practice at my own home alone.

In search of some social interaction with others, it was my choice to join a neighbour from Ashtead who was attending an over fifty five Tai Chi class on Mondays. Desperate measures were required. My only problem was I was under fifty five. A little problem I would overcome, lying about my age worked when I was a ski instructor in Scotland at the grand age of fifteen and the year later working in Italy, it was going to be a doddle to get into a Tai Chi class. Now enrolled in the class, where the average age was seventy, and the topics of conversation revolved around hospital appointments and hearing aids, this was extremely entertaining, a light relief and great distraction from my own concerns. I looked forward to this on a weekly basis at the time.

In the October of 2013, 8 months after surgery, after regaining some movement in the shoulder I took up swimming at Dorking baths. I was averaging a 20 minute swim with the focus on wishing to regain the natural movement of my right shoulder and arms where I still had some stiffness following the frozen shoulder.

My bike experience has been disappointing. When I was planning to do the Ride 100 London in July 2014, after only 11 miles out on my first session with two super fit cyclists, my energy levels went to zero in seconds. I was spent. I sent my excuses shortly afterwards to the charity organiser Alex Smith of the Harrison's Fund saying I wouldn't be able to get fit in time for the ride. I was gutted. It is my goal in 2017 to do some similar cycle distance or possibly further, I will just have to wait and see. First I will stick to cycling locally.

I knew I wanted to run, but needed to gain more stamina so had the idea that Pilates would help to increase my movement. I got a double bonus, because it also built up my stamina, a great gain.

To improve my cardiovascular function and my lung capacity I opted for a few runs, I chose to run two weeks before I went skiing. I felt this gave a chance to see if I was fit enough for my impending ski trip in the New Year and it did, but it was too soon after surgery, as it zapped my energy.

When it came to sailing, this was a no brainer. I took to doing it because being on the water takes me away from all other thoughts. I am totally focused, in a distracted way, to relax and enjoy all the elements that sailing brings to the table. Thinking of the wind, how the sails should be set, which is the fastest route in the tide and wind, and making sure the boat is balanced all the time, no focus on me, only the team work in the boat. To achieve this takes skill and a lot of concentration. I still have a long way to go to achieve this balance whilst sailing. But for now I am happy in the line up of the Flying Fifteen national championship in Hayling Bay in 2016, awesome sailing conditions a great regatta.

Skiing and sailing are my two favourite leisure activities and I was only able to do them after putting together a series of exercises to ensure I was fit enough to still hold some energy in the fuel tank. Perfect.

Stretching is something I incorporate in my daily routine and will continue to do so, to cement my core body and muscle strength.

Recognising I had to have a different mental approach

Enjoying the rewards of the little wins

Understand it great to do it for myself

The goal setting kept me focused and made it achievable

How do I feel from doing this exercise?

After the first frozen shoulder in 2013, I would have answered this question differently. Now I have nothing to prove, other than enjoy the experience. I opted on the side of caution rather than to push ahead, and continue with this attitude even now. It don't do exercise to prove to others I am well, I do it because I like to, it is my choice. These are the definite benefits of doing exercise, call it what you will. I just like doing different things, it is invigorating having time to do all these different activities, allow me to

Feel energised

Feel motivated and refreshed

In good health, working towards perfect wellbeing

I am in a more relaxed state of mind

Feel comfortable with my future goals I have set

Happy with what I have achieved to date, without busting a gut

Be ready and relaxed for what is ahead

Little did I know that exercise I was doing was allowing me to gain more stamina, thou reducing my tiredness ultimately. Let me share what I thought was acceptable state to be in the coming chapters.

Chapter 15:
Recognising the difference in fatigue or tiredness

"It took a long time for me to stop, listen and relax to my body tell tale signs."

My life was very busy, I came across for years strong and able to keep going, never stopping to rest, or stopping to listen to my body. OK I learnt techniques to put energy in me by meditating for work and leisure. Sometimes meditation was a useful technique, but not always. Now I do meditation to relax and let nature take its course. I felt if I kept going I would be fine and tiredness would be replaced once I put refreshing new experiences and activities in its place. So wrong what I learnt recently was when I feel tired I stop. It is not rocket science. Time to rest, take time to give my body space to recover and gain energy once again naturally. These days I am not shy of going to bed before 7 at night, and happy to have sofa days. Far from being lazy, 5 months post surgery, to relax it is a great feeling spending time on the sofa.

Questions
Here is an example of how I continued to work through fatigue?

I am not sure now, knowing what I am about to write, whether this is the normal level of work expected on a daily basis, OK there are a few sectors who do this level of work, these can include people from the emergency services, operational teams and crazy me to.

When I first started up my business, as it was growing it was my choice, I knew no different; in the coming pages I will demonstrate how far I pushed myself in continuing to work even though my tiredness took me to a state of fatigue.

This is an example of what I thought it was acceptable to put my body and mind though to undertake and complete a project. When asked by the client initially I had reservations about the project, so I did know the project came with some gaps. I was equally excited to be offered the opportunity in 2000, as their company was going through a big restructure of growth, their business at the time had gaps in the processes which I found out much later to my detriment. The company today and rightly so, is a well respected and extremely successful global organisation.

Let me set the scene. A member from the admin team contacted me. They had already confirmed the hotel in Madrid and appointed their production team from old to assist. My role initially was to source a venue for their final night gala dinner for about 250 guests. I took the admin lady for a site inspection to view the dinner venue, whilst there we also visited the main conference hotel. On my return I reported my findings to the Sales

Director, looking at how I saw the event working, with some problems. From this meeting I was handed the baton to manage the event from the registration, bedroom allocation and catering, plus arrange some extra entertainment on the first night of the conference as well as still manage the gala dinner. He later requested I took over the transfers to and from the airport and various hotels drop-off daily, and source interpreters for the Japanese delegation.

With the event less than 2 months away I was working with their administrator in the Chertsey office checking over the details in readiness for the delegate packs for the attendees, the various workshops, flights, special requirements etc., By less than a few weeks to go the event numbers swelled to nearer the 500 mark, by the week before we were hitting 600 plus mark. Alarm bells were ringing. I spoke with the director, concerned about the sizes of the breakout rooms allocated. He assured me the production team had it all in hand.

The week prior to the event, faced with swelling numbers, co-ordinating multiple flight pick-ups, hotel transfers and daily transfers, and needing to book extra bedrooms, I was becoming time shy and needing to work many long hours. Fortunately with my tour operator experience working at Thomsons in the winter of 1991/2 I was fine with multiple transfers and pick ups from the airport totalling 14 individuals daily. On top of the airport arrivals and departure transport. I found this relatively easy as I simplified the process by notifying the delegates in the form of a booklet that could be duplicated and given out or displayed at the various hotels with key information, times of pick-ups, updates, changes and agenda. The pressure was on to get the bedrooms correctly allocated at the right hotels, prior to booking the transport or preparing the packs.

Now in Madrid 2 days before the conference commenced, with increasing demands on my resources, I had to arrange for a gift to be placed in each of the guest's bedrooms before they checked in. The consignment arrived at the main hotel, these had to be counted sorted and couriered to the various hotels with a rooming list confirming which room each gift had to go in. The company having failed to take up sole occupancy of any of the hotels caused extra work whereby I had to double check the room allocation on the day at each of the hotels and cross reference them doing spot checks at the same time.

Still with the final preparation not completed for the packs for the coach leaders who were going to be based at the airport, I had another late night ahead of me, addressing all the envelopes personally for each of the delegates. These were assigned by coach, flight no and time and name of delegate including any special request they had made. I was fortunate to have such great ground crew at the airport, which helped the whole process run much smoother. Now with completed packs, I was confident everything there was covered.

The Sales Director now decided he wanted every guest to be greeted on arrival at each hotel. This was difficult, well actually impossible. I did not have enough internal crew to man this, so all the welcome desks were unmanned. I tried to cover two of the satellite hotels however, the main hotel had more pressing issues to deal with.

Delegates arrived plus unexpected deliveries, causing extra demands on me. Lots of boxes arrived containing personal items for each of the goody bags. I was under the impression that everything had been sourced and sent to the Chertsey offices beforehand, oh no, how wrong was I, every country took it upon themselves to send over something to place in the goody bag thinking it was a nice idea to send them directly to Madrid rather than let me know that extra shirts, pens, pads, caps were en-route. With no time allocated to check the shipments or staff to help unpack the boxes, I pulled a few reluctant members together to help me make up the goody bags. So faced with a lack of the right quantity of merchandise some goody bags were missing an item or two. It was awful, delegates scrambling to secure their goody bag, it was a bun fight, everyone was complaining and the conference hadn't even started.

Somehow I was surprisingly alert on the conference day. Tasks included managing the welcome of the delegates and checking interpreters were in place. Presentation handouts were sorted whilst keeping check of timing of catering and the evening entertainment, with constant numbers and flight changes, the demands from 600 plus delegates was overwhelming. I had one saving grace; my ground crew fortunately were great including the team at the airport. The conference started on time on day 1 as everyone was happy to follow the smartly dressed girls with beaming smiles into the main room, who wouldn't follow them? They were a welcoming help at the time.

The interpreters were standing ready to hand out the headsets as guests were about to listen to the opening address. I had brought this team of interpreters from the UK specifically to look after the Japanese speaking delegation. The style of interpretation was designed to give them straight translation of the whole conference. However, the lead director decided to start the opening address in English without the aid of the Japanese interpreters who was standing right next to him at the front. Duh. Yes. So at lunch time I had to ask the interpreters to walk through the guests to sort out who needed assistance and handed out the head sets then, there were over 40 who didn't understand a word of the morning session. Wonderful, a comedy of errors and totally unnecessary.

There was no let up for me after lunch, the production team flagged up a big issue they were having with their projector bulbs blowing. They recognised they would not have been able to continue with back projection for the presentation for the conference if any more bulbs blew, they asked me for help. OK after a few checks we found out why the bulbs were blowing; their power supply was not stable. What happened next?

I called a meeting with the hotel Director to pin point the issue. With his team of Engineers they confirmed the hotel conference rooms were not earthed correctly, fortunately the hotel team set out to carry out the repairs by bringing in an external company to sort this out immediately. Overnight they connected a new phase 3 power source, drilling a big hole to link the power supply to the conference room with the kitchen, they even had a man scaling the outside of the hotel building to re-earth the place. At 1:30am I got to sleep.

None of this would have happened if the production team had carried out the right risk assessment in the first place, it was frustrating and annoying, as I had no control other than to sort it out when the horse had bolted.

Day 2 at the 6 am morning meeting with the hotel Director, the Engineers and Production team to verified all work had been completed and the power supply was now stable. The conference could resume on schedule. The delegates descended on the hotel from various destinations and were ushered in to the main room totally unaware of the problems over the past 20 hours.

The next mess occurred after coffee break. The conference was scheduled to split into their breakout sessions. It didn't help that some of the delegates did not go to their assigned workshop. However, I was told all would be fine. It wasn't fine, we had 20 plus delegates outside the breakout room trying to squeeze themselves into the room that was obviously too small for the number wishing to attend the session. I hated that moment, one of those "told you so" moments. I had been saying this all along. However, I was assured by the company's production team that they would fit. My opinion was received with deaf ears. The production team had the final say, they were in charge of the room layouts and they were happy with what they had planned.

More unplanned changes that afternoon and evening on top of my other tasks, I had to source and re-assign new breakout rooms and keep everyone up to date with the changes. Simple things took time like creating new signage and meeting with the interpreters to request if they would change their style of interpreting from interpreter booths to whispering interpretation. Surprisingly the interpreters were most accommodating and accepted the change with ease.

Day 3 heavy-eyed, from another night of only 4 hours sleep, because of having to juggle keeping the International conference on track due to external forces not listening in the first place, I had been prevented from doing all the things I should have done, like final checks to sort out for the gala dinner, transfers there, table numbers, timing, and speeches which I had to do while running the evening entertainment of indoor fun fair side stalls, not forgetting the final preparations for departure day and transfer notices for homeward bound flights for all delegates. Fortunately with the help of meditation using a technique learnt back in the late 70's, in the morning I came across at breakfast as bright as a button with the look of confidence that everything was sorted. It gave me amazing results at the time, those techniques kept me focused and calm. If I was honest very few individuals actually knew how much work I was doing behind the scenes, I remember when someone came up to me and asked me if I could arrange or find a cigar cutter, one of the Directors said "I think she has more important things to do." Possibly an understatement if I say so myself.

Day 4 with the conference drawing to a close and amazingly running to schedule, God only knows how, after lots of thanks, flowers, and now at the part of the day when all boxes were packed, and delegates heading off on respective coaches, I was past tidiness and looking for a place to hide and rest. I found a perfect place to relax in quietness. The ideal solution was to have my hair done. I wouldn't need to talk to anyone, physically and mentally I couldn't. More demands were put on me, I was approached just before heading off to have my hair done, if I would have a de-brief with the next year's organiser, an internal person from their organisation, right there and then. Surprisingly I said no let's do it when back in the UK. I think I came across rude. I was past caring, so tired, nothing left.

A couple of hours later on the plane bound for home, a welcome thought. I asked the air hostess if I could sit in a quiet place possibly at the back and requested she needn't wake me until we landed back in the UK. She had a discerning look at me, saying "you are looking rather pale are you alright." "Yes just tired." That was an understatement, if I say it myself on reflection, it took me weeks to recover and regain my energy but my body, bones, muscles were way beyond tiredness, they were at a stage of total fatigue. With my sugar levels dropped far too low I was admitted to hospital a few weeks later for a week's rest. All I needed was quietness, good rest and some proper food. What an unhealthy state to be in.

Fair to say I don't think they had a clue of what was expected on running an event of this size. Nor do I think they appreciated how much I was doing at the time.

What measures have I put in place to manage the sensible amount of work expected from one person, which is acceptable?

From this event I adopted a few golden rules when working on large events. I start with seeing their brief of the event. I measure up by outlining the time line for each task, as well noting the processes required to complete each task. I check every task is allocated to the right members of staff to achieve the right outcome. I check the team understand their involvement, especially if they are not my personal team members, if they are not one of my team members I check they have the right experience and skill set. Then and only then I say yes I will look after your event.

Always draw up a contract outlining each task and role, making out terms and conditions.

If working with suppliers, I like to see their method statement and risk assessments and the brief they are working from to check all the processes are put in place.

For all work and leisure commitments I check if the time on that activity is well spent and what benefits will I get from doing that task and make sure I have the right balance of energy for work, rest and play.

I will say no. I have stopped trying to play the juggling act with my life. My diary is no longer split into sections. I look at doing one things at a time rather than juggling my time. Looking to ensure I use my time to my best ability and efficiently.

BENEFITS

Few golden rules when working on large events

Outline task and roles

Check my time is well spent

Being efficient on tasks

What was the biggest plus when I learnt to retain energy and not be tired?

The great thing was my everyday life experiences come easier. I never thought that it would be possible for my mind to function better, OK, what do I mean? I still have moments of great tiredness where I become forgetful and leave things in wrong places. What I have noticed by focusing to retain my energy for me is how my English grammar seems to flow easier, very surprising. Bearing in mind my dyslexia, I can recall things easier. The proof is in the pudding they say, see what you think reading this book, so far?

The extra energy has brought me immense happiness writing this, what a shift, I see lots of good things happening in my life when in the past I only saw things that wore me down. It is incredible now feeling energised, how can I describe how it is for me? Around me I feel a positive force has engulfed me, with this new found energy it has given me lots of different options and direction to choose from in my life. In the past, I had lost my excitement, now it feels like spring with the blossoming flowers daily. I recognise what I have and value this source of energy. I am always looking at ways of retaining my daily energy source rather than giving it away.

Creating the right balance of energy for work,
rest and play

Life experiences became easier daily,
things flow natually

The extra energy has brought me immense happiness

I am excited and blossoming daily

The new experiences I have explored have brought me some great benefits. I am still uncovering something new each time I dig deeper. For me the next stone unturned I like to share now is, what would be the best way to aid my recovery quicker?

Chapter 16:
Say no with ease

"This for me was a big attitude shifter to say no. Calmness only comes when I have space, balance only happens when I recognise and I give myself space"

Learning to say no without guilt, do I mean guilt? No I felt I was coming across selfish, uncaring, a quality I didn't like in myself. It isn't an easy task at first to say no. My objective is to share how having too many things happening at once complicated my life. I believed it was good if I filled all gaps with moments, when really all I was doing was hiding from something, like worry; guilt, uncertainty. Consequently all it was doing was draining all my energy. I will explain in the coming pages how I gained a better life balance by saying no and retained, regained my energy for me.

Questions
When did I realise I had to say no?

Way back before this date of 2011 I would frequently be reminded to include no in my vocabulary. At the time in 2011, I think I missed it, as I was so fully committed looking after the presidency of the British Isles Flying Fifteen Association, enrolling in the 30 week accelerator programme KPI6, whilst in the throws' of organising the Austrian Olympic and Paralympics National house for the Corporation of Trinity House. As you can see I was being pulled in lots of different directions. How did I fit in sailing and being a loving wife? I just don't know how I did it without saying no, possibly I didn't.

My real breakthrough moment to say no with ease started when I used the word no. Let's not beat myself up, to say it took longer than it should have is an understatement. I really only introduced it when I turned fifty five. Better late than never. Everything from then on began to make sense.

Then I met Tony J. Selimi (I mentioned earlier) shortly after my lung operation in 2015, we connected via Jo Davison Blue Cow Summit. He came highly recommended. It felt like the right time to meet up to look at and explore my options. His thoughts resonated with me, I didn't realise the little word 'no' was so powerful, powerful enough that it has now given me options which I didn't have before. How did I feel?

Why did I feel guilt and selfishness?

I was on uncomfortable ground, so why would I now say no, as up to April 2015 it was my choice to normally say yes? So far as I was aware it was in my make-up to say yes, could you image how I felt suddenly saying no? Awful at first, I felt like I was letting family, friends and colleagues down. Imagine what was going on in my head and my tummy, in turmoil again.

With the u-turn from yes to no, there were times I was scared. In the period of this shift I felt I lost my self worth, I truly believed what I had been doing in the past was good so this was difficult for me to comprehend. It took some months to realise how good it was for me to say no. Plus the benefits when I appreciated there were others far more equipped to help rather than me every time. I had never been in the place before to stop and think, actually there is someone else better equipped at this moment in time to help you, rather than me. Now it did make sense.

When I initially said no I felt everyone I knew or who asked me, would think I was being selfish. I equally felt guilty even before someone asked me to do something, as I knew I was going to say no, for me it felt like I was closing the doors on them, our friendship, trust and respect. Thoughts crept in with leaps and bounds of doubt and worry engulfing my head as I felt I was letting them down in a big way.

Having this initial feeling as if I had closed the door gave me a sense of loneliness. I believed they would not wish to share their friendship or invite me to be involved when they were doing something special. I remembered my thoughts going back all those years when as a child that I spent time alone it was uncomfortable, empty. Not a place I wanted to revisit. This was all milling along in my head, along with the other things going on in my life.

How did I go about saying no?

This is how I go about saying no now. I ask myself a simple question first before making my decision.

If I say yes will it benefit me, mentally, personally or physically, is it going to save time or create a better quality of life for Peter, or others members of the family or dear friends or I? If the answer is no than I will happily say no.

There must be someone else out there more qualified to help, let me think, put them in touch and let them get on with it.

BENEFITS

By saying no, it has freed up me more time

Everything began to make sense

'No' was a powerful word

No, has given me new options

What were the consequences of saying no?

Funny, it is amazing what positive results came from saying no, here are some examples of the consequences.

I am not agonising over my decisions

It is clear to me why I said no or agreed not to do something

I am not faced with juggling my time because I said yes

I have learnt to focus on what I can do well

The time saved has enabled me to allocate the time to things I will benefit from

See the shift:

I am more inclined to meet deadlines in every aspect of my life

I have more energy to do the things I like doing

I am surprised how much free time I have

I am not agonising over things that I should be doing or thinking of an excuse why I haven't done them in the first place

It is my choice to make that shift, yes, definitely calmer in all aspects of myself and my life

I have a better quality of life

Someone else out there is more qualified to help

Happy with my decision

Definitely calmer in all aspects of myself and my life

This is another stepping stone that I uncovered. What else is preventing me from me having a more fruitful life?

Chapter 17:
Seeing the benefits of saying thank you and feeling blessed

"I have seen an incredible shift change, in my life. It is great to feel my eyes and face shine when I smile with happiness"

My idea is to share how those little words of thanks were received by others. This authentic approach comes straight from the heart. Opening up my heart has made a big difference to my life, for the good.

Questions
What was my vocabulary like in the past?

OK, I just sometimes missed the opportunity to express my gratitude. I would say please and thank you and be polite in many respects, possibly an over excited child missing the moment sometimes to express my gratitude. Not considering the need to count my blessings. Another trait of mine, to survive as the youngest of 3 girls I learnt quickly to adopt the skill of being assertive in what I wanted, so I was very clear in my actions, to get what I wanted with ease, yes a polite pushing way.

When things came my way, I felt I was the right person to be doing it at the time, never stopping to consider my thanks from the bottom of my heart. (I know I was happy and was thankful, but somehow never knew how to express it in the right words) maybe because I hadn't heard my parents express gratitude or thanks regularly in their everyday life. Don't get me wrong both my parents were not rude, nor I. If anything I was over excited and everything happened so fast, in the excitement I possibly missed the right moment to say thank you, like my parents possibly too. They are not here anymore, so they cannot comment on my theory.

I was taught and told as a child to write thank you letters. This I found a chore, rather than reflecting on how lucky I was, bearing in mind how awful I was at the command of English grammar, or the movement of the pen onto paper. If I am truly honest, at Christmas I would forget who gave me what, as my parents spoilt me rotten showering me/us with lots of presents, no individual present stood out, all of them did. It was amazing, the tree was overwhelmed with presents and bows. It took until I was fifteen when I awarded a B+ in for English homework that I realised my drawing could be just as well received as a written thank you letter. That one act by that teacher, it has been amazing. Christmas presents and cards had a different meaning from then on, I looked forward to drawing a thank you card. My whole vocabulary changed, I could express myself with a picture.

Why did I want to change my vocabulary?

I was not sure why at first this came about. It wasn't as if I didn't appreciate and wasn't polite, nor was it as if I was missing out on something. I wanted to move away from the situation where I had those "if only moments." Had I actually really thought about what I was about to say and why? Rather than just saying thank you in a passing comment as expected.

What did I do? I listened. I stopped to appreciate how it made me feel giving thanks and receiving thanks. Things changed in how I said thank you from then on.

BENEFITS

Different meaning of expressing thanks from the heart

Big difference to my life for good

I appreciated how it made me feel

What happened when I changed my vocabulary?

I felt a sense of pride in changing my vocabulary. Why was I saying it?

I saw that friends and colleagues I came into contact with valued my words. For those who know me, I am not known for being a lovey-dovey person, on the contrary, and wasn't going to become one. I happy with most of my traits, they are not going to change. I have a lot of fun being who I am. I am possibly best described as having a childish sense of humour with a bit of naivety in the mix.

I felt new channels of conversation opening up for me. Let me explain, and consider what I am about to say carefully. Not because I am unsure. But what I have to say for me is important and valuable. Remember it is still difficult for me to put everything into words. Friends and colleagues now want to listen, to hear what I have to say, this is a good feeling thank you. I feel blessed.

I find it easier finding the right vocabulary spontaneously in conversations it flows naturally in everyday situations most of the time, so I don't miss the moment. It feels great, having this new quality unlocked from me. It is my choice to feel blessed because I absolutely believe how lucky I am and want to shout out my thanks. I like myself, I like being, and I value the kindness of others.

What did I do to make this change?

Let me recap I had to listen to my heart, sharing my inner me. What was different and astonishing was the great enjoyment and warmth in the response I received with the shift in my vocabulary. I found friends or those who came my way appreciated these words, receiving the thanks and blessings from me with open arms.

Felt a sense of pride

New channels of conversation opening up

Conversations flowed naturally

I value the kindness and warmth of others

Boy, such a big shift, aren't I the luckily one. I absolutely never expected to uncover this when I started out on the journey 'to look after myself to my best ability' gosh incredible discovery. There are many more stones I would like to explore, but for the time being there is one more I would like to share with you.

Chapter 18: Realise, accept help

"It is absolutely great to say yes when someone offers help, it is a gift they want to help"

I have learnt that people love to help, and it is rewarding having others involved in some part or form. It is a nice place to be, involved in a team having fun. I now see the value in how things are created and can only grow bigger with others' involvement. You cannot be a team or a team player if you are on your own. This is what I would like to share with you, the positives of having others helping, in the coming part of this chapter.

Questions - Why did I feel it was fine to do it on my own for so long?

It was scary to put this on paper, I am sharing the inner me, my heart is pounding whilst I write this bit. Not because of worrying about your thoughts of me, but of sheer excitement that I can share these thoughts, it helps me to understand I am not alone. I hope you benefit from reading this.

I thought it was a weakness to ask for help. A good place to start explaining, possibly, is to go back to the grassroots. When I was younger, (funny how it is follows a similar pattern to all the preceding answers). I had a bad experience when my father believed he was helping me with my homework. This is what happened, when he thought he was helping me he would begin by giving me a lecture on how important it was to get it right, he never grasped or understood my situation and we would consequently end up arguing, a shouting match more out of frustration than anger. So I soon stopped asking for help.

Following on from home life, now at school I basically failed to do my homework. Not because I didn't want to do it. It was because, either I didn't understand what I had to do in the first place, or I was too scared to ask in fear of looking useless. When I did understand the home-work there was no way I could transcribe it on to paper in an articulate way, so I soon became disinterested. It was easier for me to say I hadn't done it. Detention was a regular pastime for me. I only once did my home work with the aid of a teacher who understood and asked me to draw a picture and write down key words, she invited me to talk it through with her when I handed in my home work, I got my first B+. It was amazing my fellow classmates with the teachers' help were supportive, a lovely feeling. What a shift. Those opportunities didn't come my way for another 30 plus years mainly because of my own thoughts and not asking for help. I conse-quently went on for years practicing English grammar daily a word a day. Just because I wanted to beat my demons of the past not doing my homework, and be confident when I had to stand up and read or present.

Then there was my mother. With her secretive manner about our finances she got our family into a lot of shit. Even years later us three girls or father were always left to sort it out or bail us out, I sense both father's and mother's reasoning of lack of self worth or trust rubbed off on me. So I felt it was easier to do it on my own, it was my choice for years to hide my weakness. I never asked for help to protect myself, this was my belief.

I recognise these are all excuses now with understanding. I wanted to open up new channels of support, how did I go about it?

BENEFITS

Sheer excitement of sharing these thoughts

Helped me understand I wasn't alone

Opened up new channels of support

This is what I do now if I don't know an answer to a question?

I accepted help

Asked for guidance

I trusted others to do it for me

I saw strength in the help of others

On accepting help from others how did things change for me?

Life got easier, things happened with ease. My energy levels went up. I had more fun with their help. I enjoyed being part of a team. I became more relaxed. It was great letting others help, as I didn't need to be in control. I know those who helped were pleased to feel part of what was happening. In work I saw my team beam with pride and eagerness. They thrived on being trusted, up went productivity. I felt happier and blessed for their help.

Would I like to continue this way of thinking since involving others and why?

Well that is a silly question, definitely yes.

Why would I want to go back to my old ways? This new train of thought serves me perfectly. I feel anchored with the support around me, which for me in many ways is comforting. Not wishing to repeat myself, this acceptance of help has given me a new lease of energy. I don't feel like I am dragging myself through mud every day. It is great experience being a team player, it is fun.

OK there is a serious side when working, but I believe teams can bring different qualities to the arena. Things seem more solid, more real and more effective in getting the work done. It is more enjoyable accepting help and sharing ideas, and a fun, rewarding experience.

On a personal note I feel lucky and blessed to have accepted help from lots of different sources. It is all about the mind changes that have created the biggest different to my wellbeing. I would be stupid to change my ways now. It is my choice to carry on accepting help.

My energy levels went up

I valued help

Enjoyed asking for guidance

It great, I have lost that feeling, I am dragging myself though mud

Luckily and blessed accepting help

Things will continue to evolve for me, this is not the end of my journey or my life choices. One conscious choice early on in 2014 was to have little or no sugar in my diet, hence the name of the book. I am much happier making that choice I feel better in my body, soul and mind. There are many more wins for me in writing this book most of which of them would not have been possible without the kind guidance, help and directions I received from so many, I do feel blessed. Aren't I the lucky one. I now realise that.

You might say there is no real ending to this book. Well this isn't the case. My reason for stopping here is because wholeheartedly it is the start of my next part of my journey, which I am happy to share at a later stage. For the time being this book came about initially without any hidden agenda other than the request by others, going through what I been through, suggesting that I shared my thoughts in 2014.

It was such a different story back in 2012, when I was tasked to write a book about my many years experience in the events industry whilst attending a course. Each time I tried to write that book, no words would flow onto the paper. The fingers and brain stayed distant and apart. On reflection maybe at the time my passion had diminished, or my mind was lost on other thoughts, which I did not realise at the time. It was only when I was asked by other cancer patient sufferers to share my account of the past couple of years, whilst I was discovering and exploring different life choices I opted for, did this book take shape in its current form. This coincided with my choice to make a promise to myself. 'To look after myself to my best ability.'

From writing each of the chapters I began to grasp where it all started, and realised what I wanted to change. Firstly by the way that I thought, then by my actions, which at the time were only seen as problems that were deeply fixed in my mind. I realise now these thoughts were blocking me from having a calmer life experience, such a feeble excuse, I hear myself saying now. Each stone I turned brought about some amazing results. Boy, the benefits to my life are incredible I am content for once, this is magical. It has opened new ways of thinking and learning. I discover lots of things are possible now, with the right mindset. Equally life for me is rewardingly authentic and has a purpose, again a refreshing thought. This still makes me feel excited as I was editing this page. Everything word written has come from my heart, equally I feel lucky for the amazing gift I have been given in sharing my experiences with you.

One of my readers Jill, said strangely "when reading your book it seemed like it was written by two different individuals" I was surprised by her comment. However, on reflection, even without any evidence to back what I am thinking, this style of change could be down to how my brain works when I am in the flow. Again I would be interested to hear your thoughts, is it linked to Dyslexia?

As I said earlier, my life choices haven't stopped. They have opened up many new possibilities for the future. My reasoning for sharing my personal account is for the purpose that it takes away fear and shows that you are not alone, life if full of rewarding opportunities which I have enjoyed sharing with you.

I like the place in life this book has taken me. My eyes sparkle, my hair shines and I am full of energy, yippee! I am no longer a spectator, I am happy to make things happen with my actions. I understand my life purpose.

I have a few promises to myself;

'to continue to look after myself to my best ability'

To accept help and trust others

Another promise is to see the top holistic specialists sit and work alongside the likes of top consultant to rid cancer from our modern World

Referring back to the question on page 18 (check this) what do you feel now?

What has stood out for you?

Can you see your pattern forming?

Where does it sit for you?

And, finally what would you like to change?

I wish you with all my heart, that you find the answers come simply when you listen to your self.

Special note of thanks

I would like to explain why I came to write this book and how lots of individuals have helped me make this book possible. I am writing this with heartfelt gratitude to you all.

Sarah Armstrong now lives as far away as possible, well that is great way to remain friends. She is possibly one of my oldest and dearest friends of some 45 years, who knows pretty much everything about me. During the many years she has lived in New Zealand she has gone down the path of alternative medicine and learnt the craft of cranial sacral therapy. As a Cranial Practitioner she specialises in predominately the care of babies. She is well read on the subject of cancer, the body make-up, and knows how the mind works and its ways. She has an amazing gift of listening and is totally committed in what she does. Over the past 4 years Sarah has frequently been here in the UK giving me support, or at the other end of a phone for over an hour at a time listening and giving recommendations. It has been incredible to have such a trusted friend, thank you.

Andrew Hunter, an Interfaith Healer. The information he has shared has been the best gift anyone could receive. I truly feel blessed and happy he wanted to share his findings with me; the document is a testament to his years of work. No credit for his knowledge goes to me, but I can take credit for listening and taking action on his years of hard work. I believed and still believe the time he has dedicated to helping others by sharing his years of research and hardship have paid off for the good. I am a testament to that. When I first started talking with him he was looking at avenues of talking with the Scottish Health Authorities; I truly hope that they took notice and listened to a man who knows what is right for the body. My nutrition is in a far better place than it has ever been before. Yes, it is still a balancing act but with focusing on his guidance I am living a happy life knowing I am doing the best for my body. Deepest thanks.

Daniel Priestley is the Co-founder of Dent Global (with offices in the UK, Australia, Singapore and USA). He is the author of three best sellers and a leading entrepreneurship speaker. I was fortunate to have learnt from Daniel, and I received some sound advice about why, when and how I could achieve more of my business goals. He seems to have enough passion about him to run around the World three times whilst still having fun. I've been most inspired by Daniel's Key Person of Influence Accelerator, which grew into a globally recognised entrepreneurship program in under 5 years. His wisdom has helped guide my ideas and got me to a place I can now present here today with my book. Amazing, thank you Daniel.

After first failed attempt to write back in 2012, Fiona, a reader, gave me a good piece of advice, but did I listen? Well yes I did for a while. She said, "you are far better presenting, so stick at doing just that." So I did. Her comment reminded me of Mrs Wort.

Tony J. Selimi, Human Behavior and Cognition Expert, Speaker, Educator and Internationally Author, I am delighted our paths crossed for the right reasons, in April 2015. He has uncovered answers mentally and physically I didn't believe were possible. In his presence I have cried, laughed and danced, he knows everything about me but never judges, remaining indifferent and open to lead me whilst he was showed me ways to ease my fears and pain inside. Tony has given me tools, shown me how to gain a better self balance in body and mind, he has equipped me on my journey through treatments, recovering from cancer to perfect health. He has taken me further to a place where I have a great self presence and embrace life with excitement, a wonderful feeling. It is credited to Tony who continues to share this gift in healing and creating a better place for me, or many other individuals who have been touched or guided with his healing hands and mind. I feel lucky he has chosen to share his secrets. To this day I still don't always grasp what he does, but one thing is for sure, he has given me the opportunity to embrace life fully in work rest and play. I feel blessed. Thank you, Tony Hamas day

Jessica McGregor-Johnson my adopted buddy from KPI. Wasn't I fortunate? She has this presence, knowing the right moment to give advice or lead me to the right person. There is no ego involved, a rare, quality attribute in today's society. Her insights led me to Andrew and my editor, two key influences in my life today. I value Jessica's beliefs and her friendship.

Thao Dang thaoski.com and Danielle Marchant these two lovely ladies have given me the courage to step out of my comfort zone to explore and opened up new opportunities for me. They have helped me recognise my self-worth. They had the skill to map the right energy and qualities even during my turmoil.

When it comes to medical teams, where do I start to show my gratitude? How well they worked together in providing the best care and attention to detail. There is no particular order; starting with the first team I came under, L A Kostuch-Bush GP, Mr W H Allum Consultant Surgeon, Dr M Allen Associate Specialist in Medical Oncologist, Dr Filshie's, Dr George, Miss Nicola Roche Consultant Breast Surgeon, Dr Alister Ring Consultant Medical Oncologist, Mr Simon Jordon Consultant in Thoracic Surgery, Mr Paul Harris Plastic Surgeon. The army of nurses, sisters, matrons, ward staff and members behind the scenes at The Epsom, St Helens, The Royal Marsden Sutton and Fulham, The Royal Brompton, London Clinic and Chelmsford Hospital. Boy that is a lot of resources. I was fortunate to be a private patient second time around. The commitment of each team of Hospital consultants was exemplary. I must say a special thank-you to the chef at Epsom for visiting me daily to talk over my menu plan and taking note of my requests and suggestions and Miss Nichola Roche for going that extra mile.

With Jayne, Nick and Alex, we had a scary but magical trip out to The Folly on the rib to Isle of Wight over Christmas during my first round of chemotherapy. That day I almost felt normal. When I lost my hair they created a space where I felt comfortable taking my scarf off in your company. The touches of caring for and putting Peter first as much as me, I cherished, as he needed more support. Jayne delivered tasty meals over the years that I could eat and also helped me bring this book to where it is today by proof reading the content and tiding up the grammar. Thank you for your kindness, my dearest friend from down the road at Hayling.

Sarah Speller has this knack of always smiling. Nothing really fazes her she is possibly the busiest friend I know. She is full of excitement, very seldom complains, such a positive friend with passion, who had time to make my amazing blanket, which I snuggle up to the comfort of most nights in Ashtead, what a gift. Both Sarah and Jayne were there in my darkest hours when my hair was falling out, the day I had the remainder shaved off. When I was in hospital recovering from an infection their smiles lifted my spirit, we nattered and laughed, giving me moments of normality.

Gillian Godwin for her hours of walking training, she had the amazing ability to put aside her own issues to take on the challenge of the moon walk with Jayne and Sarah in aid of breast cancer research, bless you. Gillian thank you and hugs, for many times you visited me at home or hospital, or taking me out for walks, our days out pampering ourselves, our trip to Edinburgh thank you for being there when I needed an ear.

Thank you Sue Stone, such a sensitive and kind old friend for taking as much care in looking after Peter and me. I felt honoured you visited me at Royal Brompton the flowers were amazing, your presence was enough.

Jules, well thank you for keeping my secrets and for looking after me by your healing hands of Reiki treatments and those times I highjack your Thai Chi classes in your garden.

When I was thinking of selecting my readers Kate Peters seem to appear, wasn't I the luckily one. I felt touched and blessed that Kate offered to be one of the readers, she has years of knowledge and understanding from a professional background in dyslexia of many aspects that life has impacted me. Warm, heartfelt thanks for your time and support and amazing comments about my books content, you touched my heart thank you.

How come I only have busy friends? Sue Parkin what can I say for your kindness for taking time out of your hectic global family lifestyle from Connecticut to pop in and spend time with me on more than one occasion, you spoilt me thank you.

Diana Dix for always bring on the lookout for something different I could eat and the magical hampers what lovely treats, our time sunning in cap 21. Woo, what a massage. I treasured the walks with Pollyanna her little dog, who bounces around with excitement, one of the gentlest dogs I have ever known.

Special mention to Caroline and Mike McIntyre for inviting Peter and I to your table at Christmas and for all those times you popped in to see me during my recovery. Caroline, I love and value your frankness you said "I would feel shit" and "I did." With those wise words, it gave me an idea of what to expect during my chemotherapy treatment. Caroline, for changing your name to star in the two Sue's quiz night in 2015 whilst I watched, thank you for being honest with compassion and care.

Brett and Jan, Brett, you are the most upbeat friend who knows all too well what I have been going through. Your positive approach is a credit to you, you continue to amaze me, when you say "it is only a little blip" "it is, I know." The time shared on those magical adventures are fun and crazy we look forward to many more. Every day is an adventure with you two. Brett once again thank you for giving me one of the biggest hugs and smiles, you are an inspiration.

A true delight to spend a few days with Michele Hannon who visited from Australia, one of my oldest and dearest friends who has an amazing laugh and still remembers my original duck story, (we would throw it around the office, it gave us a perfect way to vent our frustrations. I remember it created a real how hoo-ha when she wrote in my leaving card don't forget the f**k-in duck). It was lovely to spend time with Michele the week after my lung operation in 2015. We are like two excited little girls who talk for hours. Poor Peter never got a word in.

My dear neighbour and sailing friend Claire Durrant for those days out to the garden centres for tea, Claire you might just get me hooked on gardening. Between you and Cousin Sarah I must express my gratitude for giving me those impossible jigsaw puzzles; they kept my mind entertained and challenged my brain cells perfectly. Karen Stewart for those lovely chats and walks during my treatment, you ear was most timely during my mother's last days, thank you.

Bless you Sue Moss my fellow quiz master for all the fun you have brought to the table, from your infectious laugh which always made me happy, to the tale when I took you sailing, a very wet day I had! The nice thoughts of so many, Carol Leaning suggesting we went for a sail and always caring, Louise for threatening if I didn't come along for a swim in her pool, she'll not be my friend. 'I love it', your character is great and kept me positive thoroughout the treatment, hugs to you too. Then big hug to Melanie and Tony Bird for bringing the smiley face of bumble bee Beatrice to see me with teddy brown bear, and teddy blonde bear cousin of teddy brown bear, and those visits from Melanie taking time out of her hectic life style to bring some calmness and keeping me in touch with the outside world.

The past couple of years my two sisters and family have been there for me, Catherine and Michael, Gerry and Ian, you have all railed around to make this period of turmoil bearable. Catherine and Michael for doing the shopping, cleaning the house, cooking the Christmas dinner and taking me to the hospital. Gerry arranging me to come on the committee boat, introducing me to your friends, for bringing the grandsons down to see me, and driving all those miles in the process, your weekly calls were welcomed, thank you.

David and Jill, Ian and Debbie for going that extra mile in being best weekend neighbours you would want for. The fun evenings, the time spent on the Dragonfly and rib, barbecuing at Easthead, and the commitment of David in agreeing to sail with me at the Europeans, I feel blessed to have such friendship thank you. Jill special thank you for making time out of your already action packed period of your life, to find the time to feedback your comments as a one of my key readers, bless you. They really helped me reshape how I set the book out in the end.

Thelma for subscribing me to VITA and for showing me I wasn't alone, and all the prompts and checks that I was doing the right exercises and stretches, a special thank you for your comments on being one of my readers, to getting me to tweak the ending. Debbie Jarvis for taking time to check I behaved and kept well.

The tremendous support from work, clients and staff giving me encouragement and support when I was tired, allowing me to reschedule appointments that fitted around my treatment, my team of freelancers for your ability to pick up the reins and deliver events with great compassion and detail, thank you.

Karen for calling me regularly from Inverness to check how my progress, gave me comfort, knowing you were there and for travelling to Loch Fyne Oyster restaurant for lunch on that windy rainy day. Mary Doogan another caring individual friend of many for taking time out of your own busy life to help and be there for me.

So many individuals touched my heart, wasn't I the lucky one? Bless you all.

Simon and Richard for making me feel happy that I can sit back and relax knowing you are both looking after Peter behind the scenes and the compassion you showed with you time, notes, messages and presents over the past few years. I would like to send my heartfelt love to two most amazing boys.

Appendices

Draft notes on Toxins to Avoid from meeting Jane Dorey Chartered Physiotherapist, Grad Dip Phy MCSP, Stage 4 cervical cancer survivor

~~Tonix~~
Toxins to avoid.

Mineral oils < Paraffin / Petroleum

Parabens ← oestrongenic presevatives)

In Purfume   Pthalates

hair Foams   Sulphates   (Sulfate)
agents.

Use Pure botanical extracts only

Jane Dorey
Thalassotherapy and holistic Spa treatment
Hear products   Balnrobics natural Toileties &
Cosmetics.

Guerrilla warfare.
Organic Food.
no dliary .
no sugar.
          Jane Dorey
Understand the cancer at Cellular level.
Very complex body.

Instant Pause January to June 2014

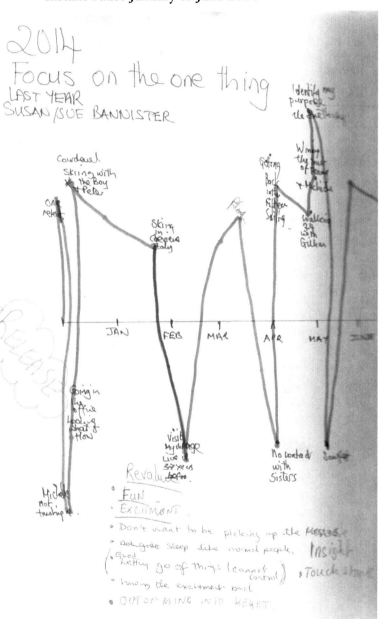

Instant Pause July to Dec 2014

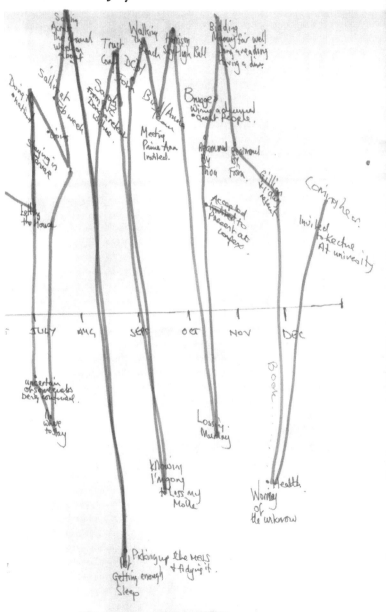

January to December 2015

You can see how balanced the year has paned out with the right focus

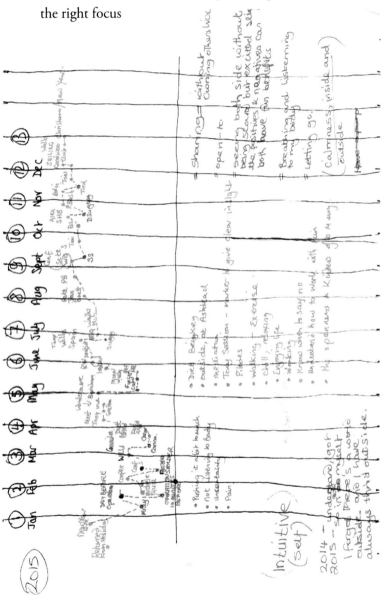

Menus

First Menu from the end of October to December 2014

	A M	MID MORN	LUNCH	DINNER
monday ①	JUICE APPLE BEETROOT CARROT	PINEAPPLE	MIXED SALAD AVOCADO LETTUCE GARLIC BEETROOT APPLE	SOUP. USE MILLET (NOT CORNFLOUR) NOT FLOUR
	BEFORE HAVE LIME/LEMON			
	~~PORRIDGE~~ PORRIDGE + COCONUT MILK			
Tuesday	JUICE SAME	PINEAPPLE	AVACADO TUNA/MAYO SALAD WITH WALNUTS + GRAPES STREWBERRIES	COD/AND BUTTER BEANS BEANS SPINACH /kale COOK WITH COCONUT OIL
	PORRIDGE + coconut			
Wednesday	JUICE SAME	PINEAPPLE	CURREY FLAVOURED MAYO WITH SALAD TOMATOET CARROT BEETROOT CHEESE.	SOUP OR SIMILAR COULIFLOUR ONION GARLIC BIT OF CHEESE PARSLEY. CHICK PEA
	PORRIDGE + coconut BLUE BERRIES			
Thursday	JUICE SAME ~~EAT~~ Lime & Lemn	BREAD SANDWICH WITH ALMOND BUTTER	ARTICHOKE Bet STEMMED CLOTH one OLIVE OIL +	SOUP OR SIMILAR FISH BAKE SWEET POTATO + BIT OF GINGER + COCONUT OIL LENTAL MILLET.
	Cucumber/Ginger water			
Friday	JUICE SAME	BANANA ~~MILK~~ + COCONUT MILK + RAW COCONUT	EGG MAYONAISE SANDWICH AND some + ALMOND Butter Sandwich	AVG CODO MAYO KALE BEETROOT BROCILI .
	Cucumber /Ginger water			
Saturday	IF HAVING JUICE RASPBERRIES STRAWBERRIES BLUE BERRIE	Apple	ROAST ~~PASTE~~ CHICKEN PESTO WITH Cauliflour.	BANANA COCONUT milk Raw. COCOA POWER
	Cucumber/Ginger Water			
Sunday	JUICE RASPBERRIE STRAWBERRIE BLUE BERRIE	Apple	Ro CHICKEN SALAD WITH CURRY MAYO + WALNUTS	BANANA COCONUT milk Raw Cocoa powder.

Menus during Chemotherapy

Day	Breakfast	Smoothie	Lunch	Dinner	
MONDAY 8AM 11	Porridge Beetroot / Tomatoes on toast	Licorice Beetroot Beans	Salad	Chicken Sausages Pineapple Tomatoes	Roast sweet potato
TUESDAY 12	Porridge	Carrot Beetroot Apple Beet Coconut	Fish Peas Potatoes Broccoli	Salmon Tomato Coconut milk	Chips SALT fat
WEDNESDAY 13	Porridge Tomatoes on toast	Carrot Beetroot Apple Coconut	Soup Butternut squash Lettuce Avocado	Not mixed Vegetable Mouthful celery that goat Bread roll	Vegetable Lettuce day soup milk
THURSDAY 14	Porridge Coconut milk	Beetroot apple Coconut	Butternut squash + celery soup	Spinach coconut milk	Cool - Poached in coconut milk
FRIDAY 15	Porridge coconut milk	Beetroot apple	Soup Vegetable (Fish + Chip) Banana	Spinach coconut milk shake	need to devise
SATURDAY 16	Porridge coconut milk	Beetroot apple coconut	Roast chicken Spinach		
SUNDAY 17	Coconut milk Blueberries Porridge	Beetroot apple Coconut	Avocado + Tomato salad Rocket (lemon/oil)	Beef Batter Cool Sweet potatoes	Christmas champagne Endive
MONDAY 18	Coconut milk Porridge coconut milk	Beetroot apple Coconut	Avocado Tomato salad Rocket + Tomato	one steamed Dates jul pork	Tongue & lentils
TREAT DAY TUESDAY 19		Beetroot apple Coconut	apple Strawberry Grapes	Soup Parsnip	
TREAT DAY WEDNESDAY 20	Strawberry Berries Smoothie		Avocado + lettuce Tomato	Courgette Leaf Bowl, Rocket Spinach Sweet potatoes Fried potatoes Eggs/Oats	Seafood Prawns / chicken Duck in Tryand Veuno Rice Pineapple Fritter

- No DIARY
- No wheat
- some meat - mainly fish (some meat)

taste buds good, can enjoy my food

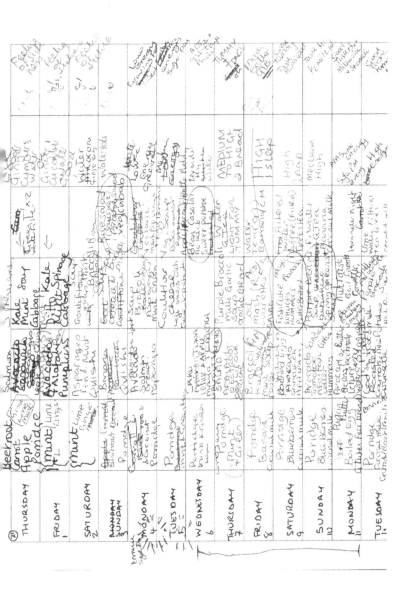

Chart monitoring body statistics during Chemotherapy

Ref to other sheet

M — SECOND PHASE of CHEMO ON (TEXOL) — S

NEXT STAGE
Temazine
Chemo — 8X
ONDANSETRON
DOMPERIDONE — 10N
DEXAMETHASONE
Neulasta injection
Pain relief
Support

Ref TEXOL
Temazine
Dexamethasone
Aqua future
Antibiotics
Pain relief
Heat
Tingly fingers
Sore feet
Clammy skin
Tingy Bum
Dehydrated
very low energy
wobbly legs

Lightning Source UK Ltd.
Milton Keynes UK
UKOW02f1040131016

285166UK00001B/7/P